THE EPI DIET FOR ENDOMORPH

A Comprehensive Guide to Balanced Nutrition, Effective Exercise, and Sustainable Wellness

Michael Luciani

Copyright © 2024

All Rights Are Reserved

The content in this book may not be reproduced, duplicated, or transferred without the express written permission of the author or publisher. Under no circumstances will the publisher or author be held liable or legally responsible for any losses, expenditures, or damages incurred directly or indirectly as a consequence of the information included in this book.

Legal Remarks

Copyright protection applies to this publication. It is only intended for personal use. No piece of this work may be modified, distributed, sold, quoted, or paraphrased without the author's or publisher's consent.

Disclaimer Statement

Please keep in mind that the contents of this booklet are meant for educational and recreational purposes. Every effort has been made to offer accurate, up-to-date, reliable, and thorough information. There are, however, no stated or implied assurances of any kind. Readers understand that the author is providing competent counsel. The content in this book originates from several sources. Please seek the opinion of a competent professional before using any of the tactics outlined in this book. By reading this book, the reader agrees that the author will not be held accountable for any direct or indirect damages resulting from the use of the information contained therein, including, but not limited to, errors, omissions, or inaccuracies.

Table of Contents

INTRODUCTION 1

UNDERSTANDING ENDOMORPH BODY TYPES 3

   Overview of the EPI Diet 3

ENDOMORPHS AND NUTRITION 6

   Characteristics of Endomorphs 6

   Importance of Nutrition for Endomorphs 7

   Common Challenges and Pitfalls 8

THE PRINCIPLES OF THE EPI DIET 10

   What is the EPI Diet? 10

   The Science Behind the EPI Diet 12

   How the EPI Diet Benefits Endomorphs? 13

CUSTOMIZING YOUR EPI DIET PLAN 16

   Assessing Your Individual Needs 16

   Setting Realistic Goals 16

   Creating a Personalized Meal Plan 17

BREAKFAST RECIPES 19

   EPI-Friendly Veggie Omelet 19

   EPI-Friendly Banana Oat Pancakes 20

   EPI-Friendly Greek Yogurt Parfait 21

   EPI-Friendly Avocado Toast 22

EPI-Friendly Berry Smoothie Bowl 23

Soothing Banana Porridge 24

Savory Spinach and Mushroom Scramble 25

Ginger Turmeric Smoothie 26

Quinoa Breakfast Bowl 27

Energizing Chia Seed Pudding 28

Hearty Quinoa Breakfast Bowl 29

Energizing Chia Seed Pudding 31

Zesty Spinach and Egg Muffins 32

Soothing Banana Porridge 33

Savory Sweet Potato Hash 34

Protein-Packed Scrambled Tofu 35

Oatmeal Breakfast Cookies 36

Egg and Veggie Breakfast Burrito 38

Creamy Coconut Chia Pudding 39

Berry Banana Smoothie Bowl 40

DESSERTS RECIPES 42

Banana Almond Chia Pudding 42

Avocado Chocolate Mousse 43

Coconut Mango Rice Pudding 44

Baked Apples with Cinnamon and Walnuts 45

Frozen Berry Yogurt Bark 46

Chia Seed Pudding with Berries 48

Baked Apple Chips 49

Coconut Banana Ice Cream 50

Chocolate Avocado Mousse 51

Cinnamon Baked Pears 52

Coconut Chia Pudding with Fresh Fruit 53

Almond Flour Banana Bread 54

Baked Coconut Mango Oatmeal Cups 56

Chocolate Peanut Butter Protein Balls 57

Apple Cinnamon Quinoa Breakfast Bars 58

Berry Avocado Parfait 60

Pumpkin Spice Chia Seed Pudding 61

Coconut Mango Rice Pudding 62

Dark Chocolate Avocado Mousse 63

Banana Oatmeal Cookies 64

SOUP RECIPES 67

Creamy Butternut Squash Soup 67

Lentil and Vegetable Soup 68

Roasted Tomato Basil Soup 70

Ginger Carrot Soup 71

- Creamy Mushroom Soup 73
- Spicy Black Bean Soup 74
- Butternut Squash Soup 76
- Lentil Soup 77
- Tomato Basil Soup 79
- Carrot Ginger Soup 80
- Spinach and Potato Soup 82
- Vegetable Quinoa Soup 83
- Creamy Cauliflower Soup 85
- Lentil and Vegetable Soup 86
- Butternut Squash Soup 88
- Tomato Basil Soup 89
- Chicken and Vegetable Soup 90
- Lentil and Spinach Soup 92
- Butternut Squash Soup 93
- Mushroom Barley Soup 95
- Tomato and White Bean Soup 96

SNACKS RECIPES 98
- Nutty Energy Bites 98
- Avocado Toast with Tomato and Basil 99
- Greek Yogurt Parfait 100

Hummus and Veggie Stuffed Pita Pockets 101

Vegetable Sushi Rolls 102

Crunchy Chickpea Snack 103

Apple and Peanut Butter Rice Cakes 104

Vegetable Crudité with Hummus 105

Quinoa and Black Bean Salad Cups 106

Banana Almond Butter Bites 107

Zesty Cucumber Hummus Cups 108

Crispy Baked Kale Chips 109

Sweet Potato Toasts with Almond Butter 110

Mango Salsa with Whole Grain Crackers 111

Quinoa-Stuffed Bell Pepper 112

Nutty Banana Oat Bars 114

Roasted Chickpea Trail Mix 115

Greek Yogurt Berry Parfait 116

Stuffed Celery Sticks 117

Turkey and Avocado Roll-Ups 118

SMOOTHIE RECIPES 120

Berry Blast Smoothie 120

Tropical Paradise Smoothie 121

Green Goddess Smoothie 121

Protein Power Smoothie 122

Coconut Kale Smoothie 123

Tropical Green Smoothie 124

Berry Spinach Smoothie 125

Creamy Avocado Smoothie 126

Peanut Butter Banana Smoothie 127

Blueberry Almond Smoothie 128

Berry Blast Smoothie 128

Green Goddess Smoothie 129

Tropical Paradise Smoothie 130

Creamy Berry Smoothie 131

Chocolate Peanut Butter Smoothie 132

Green Detox Smoothie 133

Berry Blast Smoothie 134

Tropical Paradise Smoothie 135

Creamy Peanut Butter Banana Smoothie 136

Vanilla Almond Protein Smoothie 136

SEAFOOD RECIPES 138

Grilled Lemon Herb Salmon 138

Baked Lemon Garlic Shrimp 139

Seared Scallops with Garlic Butter 140

Grilled Shrimp Skewers 141

Pan-Seared Halibut with Lemon Herb Sauce 142

Cajun Grilled Shrimp Tacos 144

Baked Lemon Garlic Cod 145

Coconut Shrimp Curry 146

Lemon Garlic Butter Scallops 148

Grilled Salmon with Dill Sauce 149

Grilled Lemon Herb Salmon 150

Lemon Garlic Shrimp Pasta 151

Baked Lemon Dill Cod 152

Garlic Butter Scallops 154

Lemon Herb Tilapia 155

Lemon Garlic Grilled Shrimp 156

Baked Salmon with Dill 157

Garlic Butter Lobster Tails 158

Tuna Salad Lettuce Wraps 159

Grilled Swordfish with Mango Salsa 160

GROCERY SHOPPING AND MEAL PREPARATION TIPS 162

Stocking Your Pantry for Success 162

Meal Prepping for Busy Endomorphs 163

Smart Shopping Strategies 165

EXERCISE AND LIFESTYLE RECOMMENDATIONS 167

Importance of Exercise for Endomorphs 167

Recommended Workouts for Endomorphs 168

Stress Management and Sleep Tips 170

MEAL PLAN 172

Day 1 172

Day 2 172

Day 3 172

Day 4 172

Day 5 172

Day 6 173

Day 7 173

Day 8 173

Day 9 173

Day 10 173

Day 11 174

Day 12 174

Day 13 174

Day 14 174

Day 15 174

Day 16 174

Day 17 175

Day 18 175

Day 19 175

Day 20 175

Day 21 175

CONCLUSION 177

INTRODUCTION

Welcome to "The EPI Diet for Endomorphs"! If you've picked up this book, chances are you're on a quest for better health and a happier relationship with your body. Well, my friend, you're in good company because I've been there, done that, and bought the t-shirt (and then had to buy a bigger size).

Let's start by addressing the elephant in the room literally, the endomorph body type. Now, if you're not quite sure what an endomorph is, don't worry, I've got you covered. Endomorphs are those of us who seem to have a genetic predisposition to hold onto every delicious calorie we consume. We're the ones who can gain weight just by *thinking* about food. If you've ever felt like your metabolism hit the snooze button while everyone else's is doing laps around the block, you're probably an endomorph. But fear not, my fellow endo-friends, this book is tailor-made for you.

So, why the EPI Diet, you ask? Well, let me tell you a little secret I've tried every diet under the sun. From the grapefruit diet to the cabbage soup diet (spoiler alert: neither involved as much grapefruit nor cabbage soup as I would have liked), I've been there, done that, and watched the scale yo-yo like it's auditioning for a circus act. But amidst the chaos of fad diets and trendy eating plans, I stumbled upon something magical the EPI Diet.

Now, I won't bore you with the science-y mumbo jumbo (unless you're into that sort of thing, in which case, I've got some extra reading material for you in the appendix), but let's just say the EPI Diet isn't just another crash-and-burn diet plan. Nope, it's a lifestyle change, a mindset shift, and dare I say, a game-changer for us endomorphs.

But before we dive headfirst into the recipes and meal plans, let's talk about something real for a moment. I get it. I understand the frustration of trying to zip up those jeans that seemed to fit just fine last week. I know the disappointment of stepping on the scale and seeing a number that makes you want to throw said scale out the window. And I definitely know the struggle of feeling like you're in a constant battle with your own body.

But here's the thing I also know that we're stronger than we give ourselves credit for. We're resilient, we're determined, and we're not afraid to tackle a challenge head-on (especially if that challenge involves a delicious plate of food). So, consider this book not just a guide to losing weight and feeling better in your own skin, but also a reminder that you're not alone in this journey.

Throughout these pages, I'll be your guide, your cheerleader, and your fellow endomorph enthusiast. We'll laugh together, we'll cook together, and most importantly, we'll support each other every step of the way. So grab your apron, sharpen your knives, and let's embark on this delicious adventure together.

Oh, and one more thing don't forget to stock up on some stretchy pants. Trust me, you're gonna need it.

Here's to good food, good friends, and a darn good life.

Cheers,

UNDERSTANDING ENDOMORPH BODY TYPES

When it comes to understanding our bodies, it's essential to recognize that we're all unique. No two individuals are exactly alike, and our bodies respond differently to various factors such as diet, exercise, and genetics. One aspect of this uniqueness lies in body types, and one such body type is the endomorph. In this chapter, we'll delve into the characteristics of endomorphs and explore how the EPI Diet can benefit individuals with this body type.

Endomorphs are one of the three primary somatotypes identified by psychologist William Sheldon in the 1940s, along with ectomorphs and mesomorphs. While everyone possesses a combination of these body types to some extent, individuals with predominant endomorphic characteristics tend to have a naturally higher body fat percentage and a tendency to store excess weight, particularly around the abdomen and hips.

Overview of the EPI Diet

The EPI Diet, short for Endomorph-Promoting Ingestion Diet, is a nutritional approach specifically designed to address the unique needs and challenges faced by endomorphs. Unlike one-size-fits-all diet plans, the EPI Diet takes into account the metabolic tendencies and dietary requirements of individuals with an endomorphic body type.

At its core, the EPI Diet emphasizes balanced nutrition, portion control, and a strategic combination of macronutrients to support weight management and overall health. Rather than resorting to extreme calorie restriction or cutting out entire food groups, the EPI Diet focuses on nourishing the body with wholesome, nutrient-dense foods while still allowing for flexibility and enjoyment in eating.

One of the key principles of the EPI Diet is the promotion of stable blood sugar levels throughout the day. Endomorphs often struggle with insulin sensitivity, which can lead to fluctuations in blood sugar levels and cravings for sugary or high-carbohydrate foods. By choosing complex carbohydrates, lean proteins, and healthy fats, the EPI Diet helps to stabilize blood sugar, reduce cravings, and promote satiety, making it easier to maintain a healthy weight.

Another fundamental aspect of the EPI Diet is its emphasis on portion control and mindful eating. Endomorphs may have a tendency to overeat or consume large portions, leading to weight gain over time. By practicing portion control and paying attention to hunger cues, individuals can learn to eat intuitively and maintain a healthy balance between energy intake and expenditure.

In addition to nutrition, the EPI Diet also incorporates lifestyle factors such as regular physical activity, adequate sleep, and stress management. These components play a crucial role in supporting metabolic health, hormone balance, and overall well-being, all of which are essential for achieving and maintaining a healthy weight.

Overall, the EPI Diet offers a sustainable and practical approach to weight management for individuals with an endomorphic body type. By focusing on balanced nutrition, portion control, and lifestyle factors, the EPI Diet empowers individuals to take control of their health and achieve their wellness goals in a way that is both effective and enjoyable. In the following chapters, we'll delve deeper into the principles of the EPI Diet and explore practical strategies for implementing it into your daily life.

ENDOMORPHS AND NUTRITION

Understanding the relationship between nutrition and body type is essential for achieving optimal health and well-being. Endomorphs, in particular, have unique nutritional needs and challenges that require special attention. In this chapter, we'll explore the characteristics of endomorphs, the importance of nutrition for this body type, and common challenges and pitfalls faced by individuals with endomorphic tendencies.

Characteristics of Endomorphs

Endomorphs are individuals who tend to have a higher percentage of body fat and a slower metabolism compared to other body types. They often have a rounded or soft appearance, with a tendency to store excess weight, especially in the abdomen, hips, and thighs. Endomorphs may also have a larger frame and find it challenging to lose weight or maintain a lean physique.

From a physiological standpoint, endomorphs typically have a lower ratio of muscle mass to body fat, which can contribute to a slower metabolism and difficulty in burning calories efficiently. Additionally, endomorphs may have a tendency to retain water and experience bloating or fluid retention, further exacerbating feelings of discomfort and dissatisfaction with their appearance.

It's important to note that while endomorphic characteristics may predispose individuals to certain challenges, they do not determine one's destiny. With the right approach to nutrition and lifestyle habits, endomorphs can achieve their health and fitness goals and feel confident in their bodies.

Importance of Nutrition for Endomorphs

Nutrition plays a crucial role in managing weight and promoting overall health, especially for individuals with an endomorphic body type. Since endomorphs have a propensity to store excess fat and struggle with weight management, adopting a balanced and nutrient-rich diet is essential for supporting metabolism, energy levels, and body composition.

One of the key principles of nutrition for endomorphs is focusing on whole, minimally processed foods that provide essential nutrients without excess calories or added sugars. This includes plenty of fruits, vegetables, lean proteins, whole grains, and healthy fats, which provide the body with the fuel it needs to function optimally without contributing to unwanted weight gain.

Endomorphs may also benefit from paying attention to their macronutrient intake, particularly the balance of carbohydrates, proteins, and fats in their diet. While carbohydrates are an important source of energy, choosing complex carbohydrates with a lower glycemic index can help stabilize blood sugar levels and prevent spikes in insulin, which can contribute to fat storage.

Protein is another crucial component of the endomorph diet, as it helps to support muscle growth and repair, boost metabolism, and promote feelings of satiety. Including lean sources of protein such as chicken, fish, tofu, and legumes in meals and snacks can help endomorphs maintain muscle mass and support their weight loss efforts.

When it comes to fats, endomorphs should focus on incorporating healthy fats such as avocados, nuts, seeds, and olive oil into their diet while limiting saturated and trans fats found in processed and fried foods. Healthy fats not only provide essential nutrients but also help to promote satiety and support hormone balance, which is important for regulating metabolism and managing weight.

In addition to choosing nutrient-dense foods, endomorphs should also pay attention to portion sizes and meal timing to support their weight loss goals. Eating smaller, more frequent meals throughout the day can help to regulate hunger hormones and prevent overeating, while also providing a steady source of energy to fuel metabolism.

Common Challenges and Pitfalls

Despite their best efforts, endomorphs may encounter various challenges and pitfalls on their journey to better health and nutrition. One common challenge is dealing with cravings for high-calorie, high-carbohydrate foods, which can derail weight loss efforts and lead to feelings of frustration and guilt.

Endomorphs may also struggle with emotional eating, using food as a coping mechanism for stress, boredom, or other emotional triggers. Learning to identify and address the underlying emotions driving these behaviors is essential for breaking free from unhealthy eating patterns and developing a healthier relationship with food.

Another challenge for endomorphs is finding the right balance between calorie intake and expenditure, especially when it comes to exercise. While regular physical activity is important for supporting metabolism and promoting weight loss, endomorphs may need to experiment with different types and intensities of exercise to find what works best for their body.

Additionally, endomorphs may face societal pressure to conform to unrealistic beauty standards and expectations, which can take a toll on their self-esteem and body image. It's important for endomorphs to focus on their own health and well-being rather than comparing themselves to others, recognizing that true beauty comes in all shapes and sizes.

In conclusion, nutrition plays a vital role in supporting the health and well-being of individuals with an endomorphic body type. By focusing on whole, nutrient-rich foods, paying attention to macronutrient balance, and addressing common challenges and pitfalls, endomorphs can achieve their health and fitness goals and feel confident in their bodies.

THE PRINCIPLES OF THE EPI DIET

Understanding the foundational principles of the EPI Diet is essential for harnessing its potential to support weight management and improve overall health, especially for individuals with an endomorphic body type. In this chapter, we'll explore what the EPI Diet is all about, delve into the science behind its effectiveness, and discuss how it specifically benefits endomorphs.

The EPI Diet, short for Endomorph-Promoting Ingestion Diet, is a nutritional approach designed to address the unique needs and challenges faced by individuals with an endomorphic body type. Unlike generic diet plans that take a one-size-fits-all approach, the EPI Diet takes into account the metabolic tendencies and dietary requirements specific to endomorphs.

At its core, the EPI Diet focuses on promoting stable blood sugar levels, supporting metabolic health, and encouraging sustainable weight loss through balanced nutrition and lifestyle habits. Rather than resorting to extreme calorie restriction or eliminating entire food groups, the EPI Diet emphasizes the importance of nourishing the body with nutrient-dense foods while still allowing for flexibility and enjoyment in eating.

What is the EPI Diet?

The EPI Diet is not a quick-fix solution or a temporary fad diet. Instead, it's a comprehensive lifestyle approach that promotes long-term changes in eating habits and behavior. The fundamental principles of the EPI Diet can be summarized as follows:

- **Balanced Nutrition**: The EPI Diet encourages a balanced intake of macronutrients, including carbohydrates, proteins, and fats, to support energy levels, metabolism, and overall health. Rather than demonizing specific food groups, the EPI Diet emphasizes the importance of choosing high-quality, nutrient-rich foods from all food groups.
- **Portion Control**: Endomorphs often struggle with overeating or consuming large portions, leading to weight gain over time. The EPI Diet promotes portion control and mindful eating, encouraging individuals to pay attention to hunger cues and eat until satisfied rather than stuffed.
- **Stable Blood Sugar Levels**: One of the key principles of the EPI Diet is stabilizing blood sugar levels throughout the day. Endomorphs may have a tendency to experience fluctuations in blood sugar, leading to cravings for sugary or high-carbohydrate foods. By choosing complex carbohydrates, lean proteins, and healthy fats, the EPI Diet helps to prevent spikes and crashes in blood sugar, reducing cravings and promoting satiety.
- **Regular Physical Activity**: While nutrition is a cornerstone of the EPI Diet, regular physical activity is also an essential component. Exercise helps to support metabolism, promote weight loss, and improve overall health and well-being. The EPI Diet encourages individuals to find enjoyable forms of physical activity and incorporate them into their daily routine.
- **Lifestyle Factors**: In addition to nutrition and exercise, the EPI Diet also emphasizes the importance of other lifestyle factors

such as adequate sleep, stress management, and hydration. These components play a crucial role in supporting metabolic health, hormone balance, and overall well-being.

In essence, the EPI Diet is not just about what you eat, but also how you eat and live. By adopting a holistic approach to nutrition and lifestyle habits, individuals can achieve sustainable weight loss and improve their overall health and quality of life.

The Science Behind the EPI Diet

The effectiveness of the EPI Diet is grounded in scientific principles related to metabolism, nutrition, and weight management. Several key factors contribute to the success of the EPI Diet in promoting sustainable weight loss and supporting metabolic health:

- **Balanced Macronutrients**: The EPI Diet emphasizes the importance of balancing macronutrients, including carbohydrates, proteins, and fats, to support metabolic function and promote satiety. Research has shown that a balanced intake of macronutrients can help regulate appetite, stabilize blood sugar levels, and support weight loss efforts.
- **Stable Blood Sugar Levels**: One of the central tenets of the EPI Diet is stabilizing blood sugar levels throughout the day. By choosing complex carbohydrates with a lower glycemic index, individuals can prevent spikes and crashes in blood sugar, reducing cravings and promoting feelings of fullness.
- **Protein-Rich Foods**: Protein is a key component of the EPI Diet, as it helps to support muscle growth and repair, boost metabolism, and promote satiety. Research has shown that a

higher protein intake can help individuals feel more satisfied after meals, leading to reduced calorie intake and greater weight loss success.

- **Portion Control**: Another important aspect of the EPI Diet is portion control and mindful eating. By paying attention to portion sizes and eating slowly, individuals can prevent overeating and reduce overall calorie intake, leading to sustainable weight loss over time.
- **Regular Physical Activity**: While nutrition is a central focus of the EPI Diet, regular physical activity is also essential for supporting metabolism, burning calories, and maintaining lean muscle mass. Research has shown that combining a healthy diet with regular exercise is the most effective approach to long-term weight management and overall health.

Overall, the science behind the EPI Diet is rooted in evidence-based principles of nutrition and metabolism. By incorporating these principles into their daily routine, individuals can achieve sustainable weight loss and improve their overall health and well-being.

How the EPI Diet Benefits Endomorphs?

Endomorphs face unique challenges when it comes to weight management, including a tendency to store excess fat and a slower metabolism. The EPI Diet is specifically designed to address these challenges and provide endomorphs with the tools and strategies they need to achieve their health and fitness goals.

One of the primary benefits of the EPI Diet for endomorphs is its emphasis on stabilizing blood sugar levels. Endomorphs may be more prone to insulin resistance and fluctuations in blood sugar, which can contribute to weight gain and difficulty losing weight. By choosing complex carbohydrates, lean proteins, and healthy fats, the EPI Diet helps to prevent spikes and crashes in blood sugar, reducing cravings and promoting feelings of fullness.

Additionally, the EPI Diet promotes a balanced intake of macronutrients, including carbohydrates, proteins, and fats, to support metabolism and promote satiety. Endomorphs may benefit from a higher protein intake, as protein helps to support muscle growth and repair, boost metabolism, and promote feelings of fullness. By including protein-rich foods in their diet, endomorphs can maintain muscle mass and support their weight loss efforts.

Portion control is another key component of the EPI Diet that benefits endomorphs. Endomorphs may have a tendency to overeat or consume large portions, leading to weight gain over time. By practicing portion control and paying attention to hunger cues, endomorphs can prevent overeating and reduce overall calorie intake, leading to sustainable weight loss over time.

In addition to nutrition, the EPI Diet also emphasizes the importance of regular physical activity for endomorphs. Exercise helps to support metabolism, burn calories, and maintain lean muscle mass, all of which are important for achieving and maintaining a healthy weight. By incorporating regular physical activity into their daily routine, endomorphs can maximize the benefits of the EPI Diet and achieve their health and fitness goals.

Overall, the EPI Diet offers a comprehensive approach to weight management and overall health that is specifically tailored to the needs of endomorphs. By focusing on balanced nutrition, portion control, and regular physical activity, endomorphs can achieve sustainable weight loss and improve their overall health and well-being.

CUSTOMIZING YOUR EPI DIET PLAN

Customizing your EPI Diet plan is essential for achieving long-term success and tailoring the approach to your individual needs and goals. In this chapter, we'll explore how to assess your individual needs, set realistic goals, and create a personalized meal plan that works for you.

Assessing Your Individual Needs

Assessing your individual needs is the first step in customizing your EPI Diet plan. This involves taking into account factors such as your age, gender, activity level, health status, and dietary preferences. By understanding your unique circumstances and requirements, you can create a plan that is both effective and sustainable.

One way to assess your individual needs is to evaluate your current dietary habits and lifestyle choices. Keep a food diary for a few days to track you're eating patterns, portion sizes, and food choices. Pay attention to how different foods make you feel and any patterns or trends you notice. This can help you identify areas for improvement and determine which aspects of the EPI Diet are most relevant to your needs.

It's also important to consider any specific health concerns or dietary restrictions you may have. If you have any underlying medical conditions or food allergies, it's essential to work with a healthcare professional or registered dietitian to ensure that your EPI Diet plan is safe and appropriate for your needs.

Setting Realistic Goals

Setting realistic goals is crucial for staying motivated and making progress towards your desired outcomes. When it comes to weight loss and improving health, it's important to set goals that are specific, measurable, achievable, relevant, and time-bound (SMART).

Start by identifying your long-term goals, such as achieving a healthy weight, improving energy levels, or reducing your risk of chronic disease. Then, break these goals down into smaller, more manageable targets that you can work towards on a daily or weekly basis.

For example, if your long-term goal is to lose 20 pounds, you might set smaller goals such as losing 1-2 pounds per week or increasing your daily physical activity. By breaking your goals down into smaller steps, you can track your progress more easily and stay motivated along the way.

It's also important to be realistic about what you can achieve within a given timeframe. Rapid weight loss may not be sustainable or healthy in the long term, so aim for slow, steady progress that you can maintain over time. Remember that progress is progress, no matter how small, and celebrate your successes along the way.

Creating a Personalized Meal Plan

Creating a personalized meal plan is the cornerstone of the EPI Diet and essential for achieving your nutrition goals. A well-balanced meal plan should include a variety of nutrient-dense foods from all food groups, including fruits, vegetables, lean proteins, whole grains, and healthy fats.

Start by determining your calorie needs based on factors such as your age, gender, weight, height, and activity level. There are many online calculators and tools available to help you estimate your calorie needs, or you can work with a registered dietitian for personalized guidance.

Once you have determined your calorie needs, you can begin planning your meals and snacks accordingly. Aim to include a balance of carbohydrates, proteins, and fats in each meal, and focus on choosing whole, minimally processed foods whenever possible.

When creating your meal plan, consider your dietary preferences, cooking skills, and lifestyle factors. If you have a busy schedule, look for quick and easy meal ideas that can be prepared in advance or made in under 30 minutes. If you enjoy cooking, experiment with new recipes and flavors to keep your meals interesting and enjoyable.

It's also important to plan for flexibility and variety in your meal plan. Don't be afraid to mix things up and try new foods, flavors, and cuisines. Including a wide range of foods in your diet not only helps to ensure that you're getting all the nutrients you need but also keeps mealtime exciting and enjoyable.

In addition to planning your meals, don't forget to plan for snacks as well. Healthy snacks can help to keep hunger at bay between meals and prevent overeating later in the day. Aim for snacks that are high in protein and fiber, such as Greek yogurt with fruit, hummus and vegetables, or a handful of nuts and seeds.

Finally, don't forget to listen to your body and adjust your meal plan as needed. If you find that you're constantly hungry or lacking energy, you may need to increase your calorie intake or adjust your macronutrient ratios. Likewise, if you're feeling satisfied and energized, you may be on the right track.

Overall, creating a personalized meal plan is key to success on the EPI Diet. By assessing your individual needs, setting realistic goals, and planning your meals accordingly, you can achieve your nutrition goals and improve your overall health and well-being.

BREAKFAST RECIPES

EPI-Friendly Veggie Omelet

Prep Time: 10 mins

Total Time: 15 mins

Servings: 2 servings

Ingredients:

- 4 large eggs
- 1/4 cup chopped bell peppers (any color)
- 1/4 cup diced tomatoes
- 1/4 cup chopped spinach
- 1/4 cup diced mushrooms
- Salt and pepper to taste
- 2 teaspoons olive oil

Directions:

1. In a bowl, beat the eggs until well combined. Season with salt and pepper.
2. Heat 1 teaspoon of olive oil in a non-stick skillet over medium heat.
3. Add the chopped vegetables to the skillet and cook for 2-3 minutes until they begin to soften.
4. Pour the beaten eggs over the vegetables, tilting the skillet to spread them evenly.
5. Cook for 3-4 minutes, or until the eggs are set around the edges.
6. Using a spatula, gently fold the omelet in half and cook for another 1-2 minutes until the eggs are fully cooked.

7. Repeat the process to make the second omelet.
8. Serve hot with a side of whole grain toast or fresh fruit.

Nutrition Facts (per serving):
- Calories: 180
- Protein: 13g
- Fat: 12g
- Carbohydrates: 5g
- Fiber: 2g

EPI-Friendly Banana Oat Pancakes

Prep Time: 5 mins

Total Time: 15 mins

Servings: 2 servings

Ingredients:
- 1 ripe banana, mashed
- 2 large eggs
- 1/2 cup rolled oats
- 1/4 teaspoon cinnamon
- 1/4 teaspoon vanilla extract
- 1/4 cup fresh berries (optional, for topping)
- Maple syrup or honey (optional, for drizzling)

Directions:
1. In a mixing bowl, combine the mashed banana, eggs, rolled oats, cinnamon, and vanilla extract. Mix until well combined.
2. Heat a non-stick skillet or griddle over medium heat and lightly grease with cooking spray or oil.

3. Pour about 1/4 cup of the pancake batter onto the skillet for each pancake.
4. Cook for 2-3 minutes on one side, or until bubbles form on the surface.
5. Flip the pancakes and cook for another 1-2 minutes on the other side, until golden brown and cooked through.
6. Repeat with the remaining batter.
7. Serve the pancakes topped with fresh berries and a drizzle of maple syrup or honey, if desired.

Nutrition Facts (per serving):
- Calories: 220
- Protein: 9g
- Fat: 7g
- Carbohydrates: 32g
- Fiber: 4g

EPI-Friendly Greek Yogurt Parfait

Prep Time: 5 mins

Total Time: 5 mins

Servings: 1 serving

Ingredients:
- 1/2 cup plain Greek yogurt
- 1/4 cup granola (choose a low-sugar option)
- 1/4 cup mixed berries (such as strawberries, blueberries, raspberries)
- 1 tablespoon honey or maple syrup (optional)

Directions:

1. In a glass or bowl, layer the Greek yogurt, granola, and mixed berries.
2. Drizzle with honey or maple syrup, if desired.
3. Serve immediately and enjoy!

Nutrition Facts (per serving):

- Calories: 250
- Protein: 18g
- Fat: 6g
- Carbohydrates: 33g
- Fiber: 5g

EPI-Friendly Avocado Toast

Prep Time: 5 mins

Total Time: 10 mins

Servings: 1 serving

Ingredients:

- 1 slice whole grain bread, toasted
- 1/2 ripe avocado
- 1/4 teaspoon red pepper flakes (optional)
- 1 teaspoon lemon juice
- Salt and pepper to taste

Directions:

1. Mash the avocado in a small bowl with a fork until smooth.
2. Stir in the lemon juice, red pepper flakes (if using), salt, and pepper.
3. Spread the mashed avocado mixture evenly onto the toasted bread.

4. Serve immediately and enjoy!

Nutrition Facts (per serving):

- Calories: 180
- Protein: 4g
- Fat: 10g
- Carbohydrates: 20g
- Fiber: 6g

EPI-Friendly Berry Smoothie Bowl

Prep Time: 5 mins

Total Time: 5 mins

Servings: 1 serving

Ingredients:

- 1/2 cup frozen mixed berries (such as strawberries, blueberries, raspberries)
- 1/2 ripe banana
- 1/2 cup plain Greek yogurt
- 1/4 cup almond milk (or any milk of your choice)
- 1 tablespoon chia seeds
- 1 tablespoon honey or maple syrup (optional)
- Toppings: sliced banana, fresh berries, granola, shredded coconut

Directions:

1. In a blender, combine the frozen berries, banana, Greek yogurt, almond milk, chia seeds, and honey or maple syrup (if using).
2. Blend until smooth and creamy, adding more almond milk if needed to reach your desired consistency.

3. Pour the smoothie into a bowl and top with sliced banana, fresh berries, granola, and shredded coconut.
4. Serve immediately and enjoy!

Nutrition Facts (per serving):
- Calories: 280
- Protein: 15g
- Fat: 8g
- Carbohydrates: 40g
- Fiber: 9g

Soothing Banana Porridge

Prep Time: 5 mins

Total Time: 10 mins

Servings: 2

Ingredients:
- 1 ripe banana, mashed
- 1 cup rolled oats
- 2 cups water or almond milk
- 1/2 teaspoon cinnamon
- Pinch of salt
- 1 tablespoon honey or maple syrup (optional)
- Fresh berries or sliced banana for topping

Directions:
1. In a saucepan, combine the mashed banana, rolled oats, water or almond milk, cinnamon, and salt.

2. Bring to a boil over medium-high heat, then reduce the heat to low and simmer for 5-7 minutes, stirring occasionally, until the oats are cooked and the mixture has thickened.
3. Remove from heat and stir in the honey or maple syrup, if using.
4. Divide the porridge into bowls and top with fresh berries or sliced banana.
5. Serve warm and enjoy!

Nutrition Facts (per serving):
- Calories: 210
- Protein: 5g
- Fat: 2g
- Carbohydrates: 44g
- Fiber: 6g

Savory Spinach and Mushroom Scramble

Prep Time: 5 mins

Total Time: 10 mins

Servings: 2

Ingredients:
- 4 large eggs
- 1 cup chopped spinach
- 1/2 cup sliced mushrooms
- 1/4 cup diced onion
- 1 tablespoon olive oil
- Salt and pepper to taste
- Fresh herbs (such as parsley or chives) for garnish

Directions:
1. In a bowl, whisk the eggs until well combined. Season with salt and pepper.
2. Heat the olive oil in a skillet over medium heat.
3. Add the diced onion and cook for 2-3 minutes until softened.
4. Add the sliced mushrooms to the skillet and cook for another 2-3 minutes until they begin to brown.
5. Add the chopped spinach to the skillet and cook for 1-2 minutes until wilted.
6. Pour the beaten eggs into the skillet and cook, stirring gently, until the eggs are scrambled and cooked to your desired consistency.
7. Divide the scramble onto plates and garnish with fresh herbs.
8. Serve hot and enjoy!

Nutrition Facts (per serving):
- Calories: 180
- Protein: 12g
- Fat: 13g
- Carbohydrates: 5g
- Fiber: 2g

Ginger Turmeric Smoothie

Prep Time: 5 mins

Total Time: 5 mins

Servings: 2

Ingredients:
- 1 cup frozen mango chunks

- 1 ripe banana
- 1 cup coconut water or almond milk
- 1/2 teaspoon grated fresh ginger
- 1/2 teaspoon ground turmeric
- 1 tablespoon honey or maple syrup (optional)
- Pinch of black pepper (to activate turmeric)

Directions:

1. In a blender, combine the frozen mango chunks, banana, coconut water or almond milk, grated ginger, ground turmeric, honey or maple syrup (if using), and black pepper.
2. Blend until smooth and creamy.
3. Pour into glasses and serve immediately.
4. Enjoy the refreshing and anti-inflammatory benefits of this vibrant smoothie!

Nutrition Facts (per serving):

- Calories: 150
- Protein: 2g
- Fat: 1g
- Carbohydrates: 37g
- Fiber: 4g

Quinoa Breakfast Bowl

Prep Time: 5 mins

Total Time: 20 mins

Servings: 2

Ingredients:

- 1/2 cup quinoa, rinsed

- 1 cup water or almond milk
- 1/2 teaspoon cinnamon
- 1 tablespoon honey or maple syrup (optional)
- 1/4 cup chopped nuts (such as almonds, walnuts, or pecans)
- 1/4 cup dried fruit (such as raisins, cranberries, or apricots)
- Fresh berries or sliced banana for topping

Directions:

1. In a saucepan, combine the quinoa, water or almond milk, cinnamon, and honey or maple syrup (if using).
2. Bring to a boil over medium-high heat, then reduce the heat to low and simmer for 15-20 minutes, or until the quinoa is cooked and the liquid has been absorbed.
3. Fluff the quinoa with a fork and divide it into bowls.
4. Top with chopped nuts, dried fruit, and fresh berries or sliced banana.
5. Serve warm and enjoy this hearty and nutritious breakfast bowl!

Nutrition Facts (per serving):

- Calories: 280
- Protein: 9g
- Fat: 8g
- Carbohydrates: 47g
- Fiber: 6g

Energizing Chia Seed Pudding

Prep Time: 5 mins

Total Time: 2 hours 5 mins (includes chilling time)

Servings: 2

Ingredients:
- 1/4 cup chia seeds
- 1 cup almond milk or coconut milk
- 1 tablespoon honey or maple syrup
- 1/2 teaspoon vanilla extract
- Fresh fruit for topping (such as berries, sliced banana, or kiwi)

Directions:
1. In a mixing bowl, combine the chia seeds, almond milk or coconut milk, honey or maple syrup, and vanilla extract.
2. Whisk together until well combined.
3. Cover the bowl and refrigerate for at least 2 hours, or preferably overnight, to allow the chia seeds to thicken and absorb the liquid.
4. Stir the pudding well before serving to ensure a smooth consistency.
5. Divide the chia seed pudding into serving glasses or bowls.
6. Top with fresh fruit and enjoy this nutrient-rich and energizing breakfast treat!

Nutrition Facts (per serving):
- Calories: 150
- Protein: 4g
- Fat: 7g
- Carbohydrates: 18g
- Fiber: 9g

Hearty Quinoa Breakfast Bowl

Prep Time: 5 mins

Total Time: 20 mins

Servings: 2

Ingredients:

- 1/2 cup quinoa, rinsed
- 1 cup water or almond milk
- 1/2 teaspoon cinnamon
- 1 tablespoon honey or maple syrup (optional)
- 1/4 cup chopped nuts (such as almonds, walnuts, or pecans)
- 1/4 cup dried fruit (such as raisins, cranberries, or apricots)
- Fresh berries or sliced banana for topping

Directions:

1. In a saucepan, combine the quinoa, water or almond milk, cinnamon, and honey or maple syrup (if using).
2. Bring to a boil over medium-high heat, then reduce the heat to low and simmer for 15-20 minutes, or until the quinoa is cooked and the liquid has been absorbed.
3. Fluff the quinoa with a fork and divide it into bowls.
4. Top with chopped nuts, dried fruit, and fresh berries or sliced banana.
5. Serve warm and enjoy this hearty and nutritious breakfast bowl!

Nutrition Facts (per serving):

- Calories: 280
- Protein: 9g
- Fat: 8g
- Carbohydrates: 47g

- Fiber: 6g

Energizing Chia Seed Pudding

Prep Time: 5 mins

Total Time: 2 hours 5 mins (includes chilling time)

Servings: 2

Ingredients:
- 1/4 cup chia seeds
- 1 cup almond milk or coconut milk
- 1 tablespoon honey or maple syrup
- 1/2 teaspoon vanilla extract
- Fresh fruit for topping (such as berries, sliced banana, or kiwi)

Directions:
1. In a mixing bowl, combine the chia seeds, almond milk or coconut milk, honey or maple syrup, and vanilla extract.
2. Whisk together until well combined.
3. Cover the bowl and refrigerate for at least 2 hours, or preferably overnight, to allow the chia seeds to thicken and absorb the liquid.
4. Stir the pudding well before serving to ensure a smooth consistency.
5. Divide the chia seed pudding into serving glasses or bowls.
6. Top with fresh fruit and enjoy this nutrient-rich and energizing breakfast treat!

Nutrition Facts (per serving):
- Calories: 150
- Protein: 4g

- Fat: 7g
- Carbohydrates: 18g
- Fiber: 9g

Zesty Spinach and Egg Muffins

Prep Time: 10 mins

Total Time: 25 mins

Servings: 4

Ingredients:

- 4 large eggs
- 1 cup chopped spinach
- 1/4 cup diced tomatoes
- 1/4 cup diced bell peppers
- 1/4 cup shredded cheddar cheese
- Salt and pepper to taste

Directions:

1. Preheat the oven to 350°F (175°C). Grease a muffin tin with cooking spray or line with paper liners.
2. In a mixing bowl, whisk the eggs until well beaten. Season with salt and pepper.
3. Stir in the chopped spinach, diced tomatoes, diced bell peppers, and shredded cheddar cheese.
4. Divide the egg mixture evenly among the muffin cups.
5. Bake for 15-20 minutes, or until the egg muffins are set and lightly golden on top.
6. Allow the muffins to cool slightly before serving.

7. Enjoy these flavorful and protein-packed egg muffins as a satisfying breakfast option!

Nutrition Facts (per serving - 2 muffins):
- Calories: 180
- Protein: 12g
- Fat: 11g
- Carbohydrates: 6g
- Fiber: 2g

Soothing Banana Porridge

Prep Time: 5 mins

Total Time: 10 mins

Servings: 2

Ingredients:
- 1 ripe banana, mashed
- 1 cup rolled oats
- 2 cups water or almond milk
- 1/2 teaspoon cinnamon
- Pinch of salt
- 1 tablespoon honey or maple syrup (optional)
- Fresh berries or sliced banana for topping

Directions:
1. In a saucepan, combine the mashed banana, rolled oats, water or almond milk, cinnamon, and salt.
2. Bring to a boil over medium-high heat, then reduce the heat to low and simmer for 5-7 minutes, stirring occasionally, until the oats are cooked and the mixture has thickened.

3. Remove from heat and stir in the honey or maple syrup, if using.
4. Divide the porridge into bowls and top with fresh berries or sliced banana.
5. Serve warm and enjoy!

Nutrition Facts (per serving):

- Calories: 210
- Protein: 5g
- Fat: 2g
- Carbohydrates: 44g
- Fiber: 6g

Savory Sweet Potato Hash

Prep Time: 10 mins

Total Time: 25 mins

Servings: 2

Ingredients:

- 1 large sweet potato, peeled and diced
- 1/2 onion, diced
- 1 bell pepper, diced
- 2 cloves garlic, minced
- 2 tablespoons olive oil
- Salt and pepper to taste
- 2 eggs (optional)
- Fresh parsley or cilantro for garnish

Directions:

1. Heat olive oil in a large skillet over medium heat.

2. Add diced sweet potato to the skillet and cook for about 5 minutes, stirring occasionally, until they begin to soften.
3. Add diced onion, bell pepper, and minced garlic to the skillet. Cook for an additional 7-8 minutes, or until the vegetables are tender and slightly caramelized.
4. Season with salt and pepper to taste.
5. If desired, create wells in the hash and crack eggs into each well. Cover the skillet and cook for 3-4 minutes, or until the eggs are cooked to your liking.
6. Garnish with fresh parsley or cilantro before serving.
7. Serve hot and enjoy this satisfying and nutrient-rich breakfast!

Nutrition Facts (per serving without eggs):
- Calories: 250
- Protein: 4g
- Fat: 14g
- Carbohydrates: 29g
- Fiber: 5g

Protein-Packed Scrambled Tofu

Prep Time: 10 mins

Total Time: 15 mins

Servings: 2

Ingredients:
- 1 block (14 oz) firm tofu, drained and crumbled
- 1 tablespoon olive oil
- 1/2 onion, diced
- 1 bell pepper, diced

- 1 cup spinach, chopped
- 2 tablespoons nutritional yeast
- 1/2 teaspoon turmeric powder
- Salt and pepper to taste
- Fresh parsley for garnish

Directions:

1. Heat olive oil in a skillet over medium heat.
2. Add diced onion and bell pepper to the skillet. Cook for 3-4 minutes until softened.
3. Add crumbled tofu to the skillet along with nutritional yeast, turmeric powder, salt, and pepper. Stir well to combine.
4. Cook for another 5-7 minutes, stirring occasionally, until the tofu is heated through and slightly browned.
5. Add chopped spinach to the skillet and cook for an additional 2 minutes until wilted.
6. Garnish with fresh parsley before serving.
7. Enjoy this protein-packed and flavorful breakfast option!

Nutrition Facts (per serving):

- Calories: 220
- Protein: 18g
- Fat: 13g
- Carbohydrates: 10g
- Fiber: 3g

Oatmeal Breakfast Cookies

Prep Time: 10 mins

Total Time: 20 mins

Servings: 8 cookies

Ingredients:

- 1 ripe banana, mashed
- 1/4 cup almond butter
- 1/4 cup honey or maple syrup
- 1 cup rolled oats
- 1/4 cup chopped nuts (such as almonds, walnuts, or pecans)
- 1/4 cup dried fruit (such as raisins, cranberries, or apricots)
- 1/2 teaspoon cinnamon
- Pinch of salt

Directions:

1. Preheat the oven to 350°F (175°C). Line a baking sheet with parchment paper.
2. In a mixing bowl, combine the mashed banana, almond butter, and honey or maple syrup.
3. Stir in the rolled oats, chopped nuts, dried fruit, cinnamon, and salt until well combined.
4. Scoop spoonfuls of the dough onto the prepared baking sheet and flatten slightly with the back of a spoon.
5. Bake for 12-15 minutes, or until the cookies are golden brown around the edges.
6. Remove from the oven and let cool on the baking sheet for 5 minutes before transferring to a wire rack to cool completely.

7. Enjoy these wholesome oatmeal breakfast cookies as a convenient and satisfying grab-and-go option!

Nutrition Facts (per serving - 1 cookie):
- Calories: 150
- Protein: 4g
- Fat: 8g
- Carbohydrates: 18g
- Fiber: 2g

Egg and Veggie Breakfast Burrito

Prep Time: 10 mins

Total Time: 15 mins

Servings: 2

Ingredients:
- 4 large eggs
- 1/2 bell pepper, diced
- 1/2 onion, diced
- 1/2 cup black beans, drained and rinsed
- 1/4 cup shredded cheddar cheese
- 2 whole grain tortillas
- Salt and pepper to taste
- Salsa and avocado slices for serving (optional)

Directions:
1. In a skillet, heat olive oil over medium heat. Add diced bell pepper and onion, sauté until softened, about 3-4 minutes.

2. Crack eggs into the skillet, scramble until cooked through, then mix in black beans and shredded cheddar cheese. Season with salt and pepper to taste.
3. Warm tortillas in a separate skillet or microwave.
4. Divide the egg and veggie mixture evenly between the tortillas, then fold into burritos.
5. Serve with salsa and avocado slices on the side, if desired.
6. Enjoy this hearty and satisfying breakfast burrito!

Nutrition Facts (per serving):

- Calories: 350
- Protein: 20g
- Fat: 15g
- Carbohydrates: 30g
- Fiber: 8g

Creamy Coconut Chia Pudding

Prep Time: 5 mins

Total Time: 2 hours 5 mins (includes chilling time)

Servings: 2

Ingredients:

- 1/4 cup chia seeds
- 1 cup coconut milk
- 1 tablespoon honey or maple syrup
- 1/2 teaspoon vanilla extract
- Fresh fruit for topping (such as berries, sliced banana, or mango)

Directions:

1. In a mixing bowl, combine the chia seeds, coconut milk, honey or maple syrup, and vanilla extract.
2. Whisk together until well combined.
3. Cover the bowl and refrigerate for at least 2 hours, or preferably overnight, to allow the chia seeds to thicken and absorb the liquid.
4. Stir the pudding well before serving to ensure a smooth consistency.
5. Divide the chia seed pudding into serving glasses or bowls.
6. Top with fresh fruit and enjoy this creamy and satisfying breakfast treat!

Nutrition Facts (per serving):
- Calories: 230
- Protein: 5g
- Fat: 17g
- Carbohydrates: 17g
- Fiber: 9g

Berry Banana Smoothie Bowl

Prep Time: 5 mins

Total Time: 5 mins

Servings: 2

Ingredients:
- 1 ripe banana
- 1 cup frozen mixed berries (such as strawberries, blueberries, raspberries)
- 1/2 cup plain Greek yogurt

- 1/4 cup almond milk or coconut water
- 1 tablespoon chia seeds
- 1 tablespoon honey or maple syrup (optional)
- Toppings: sliced banana, fresh berries, granola, shredded coconut

Directions:

1. In a blender, combine the ripe banana, frozen mixed berries, Greek yogurt, almond milk or coconut water, chia seeds, and honey or maple syrup (if using).
2. Blend until smooth and creamy, adding more almond milk or coconut water if needed to reach your desired consistency.
3. Pour the smoothie into bowls.
4. Top with sliced banana, fresh berries, granola, and shredded coconut.
5. Serve immediately and enjoy this refreshing and nutritious smoothie bowl!

Nutrition Facts (per serving):

- Calories: 250
- Protein: 9g
- Fat: 7g
- Carbohydrates: 40g
- Fiber: 9g

DESSERTS RECIPES

Banana Almond Chia Pudding

Prep Time: 5 mins

Total Time: 2 hrs 5 mins

Servings: 2

Ingredients:

- 1 ripe banana
- 1 cup almond milk
- 1/4 cup chia seeds
- 1 tablespoon honey or maple syrup
- 1/4 teaspoon vanilla extract
- Optional toppings: sliced almonds, fresh berries

Directions:

1. In a blender, combine the ripe banana, almond milk, honey or maple syrup, and vanilla extract. Blend until smooth.
2. Transfer the banana mixture to a bowl or jar.
3. Stir in the chia seeds until well combined.
4. Cover and refrigerate for at least 2 hours, or until the chia pudding has thickened.
5. Once thickened, stir the chia pudding to evenly distribute the seeds.
6. Serve the chia pudding topped with sliced almonds and fresh berries, if desired.
7. Enjoy this creamy and nutritious banana almond chia pudding as a satisfying dessert or snack!

Nutrition Facts (per serving):
- Calories: 200
- Protein: 5g
- Fat: 8g
- Carbohydrates: 30g
- Fiber: 10g

Avocado Chocolate Mousse

Prep Time: 10 mins

Total Time: 10 mins

Servings: 2

Ingredients:
- 1 ripe avocado
- 2 tablespoons cocoa powder
- 2 tablespoons honey or maple syrup
- 1/4 teaspoon vanilla extract
- Pinch of salt
- Optional toppings: sliced strawberries, shaved dark chocolate

Directions:
1. Scoop the flesh of the ripe avocado into a blender or food processor.
2. Add the cocoa powder, honey or maple syrup, vanilla extract, and a pinch of salt.
3. Blend until smooth and creamy, scraping down the sides as needed.
4. Divide the avocado chocolate mousse into serving glasses.

5. Refrigerate for at least 30 minutes before serving to allow the mousse to set.
6. Serve topped with sliced strawberries and shaved dark chocolate, if desired.
7. Enjoy this rich and indulgent avocado chocolate mousse as a guilt-free dessert option!

Nutrition Facts (per serving):
- Calories: 180
- Protein: 3g
- Fat: 12g
- Carbohydrates: 20g
- Fiber: 7g

Coconut Mango Rice Pudding

Prep Time: 5 mins
Total Time: 25 mins
Servings: 2

Ingredients:
- 1/2 cup cooked rice (such as basmati or jasmine)
- 1 cup coconut milk
- 1 ripe mango, diced
- 2 tablespoons honey or maple syrup
- 1/4 teaspoon vanilla extract
- Pinch of cinnamon
- Optional toppings: toasted coconut flakes, chopped nuts

Directions:
1. In a saucepan, combine the cooked rice and coconut milk.

2. Bring to a simmer over medium heat, stirring occasionally.
3. Once simmering, reduce the heat to low and continue to cook for 15-20 minutes, or until the rice has absorbed the coconut milk and the mixture has thickened.
4. Remove from heat and stir in the diced mango, honey or maple syrup, vanilla extract, and a pinch of cinnamon.
5. Divide the coconut mango rice pudding into serving bowls.
6. Serve warm or chilled, topped with toasted coconut flakes and chopped nuts, if desired.
7. Enjoy this tropical and comforting coconut mango rice pudding as a delightful dessert or snack!

Nutrition Facts (per serving):
- Calories: 250
- Protein: 3g
- Fat: 10g
- Carbohydrates: 40g
- Fiber: 4g

Baked Apples with Cinnamon and Walnuts

Prep Time: 10 mins

Total Time: 40 mins

Servings: 2

Ingredients:
- 2 apples (such as Granny Smith or Honey crisp)
- 2 tablespoons chopped walnuts
- 1 tablespoon honey or maple syrup
- 1/2 teaspoon cinnamon

- Pinch of nutmeg
- 1/4 cup water

Directions:

1. Preheat the oven to 375°F (190°C). Grease a baking dish with non-stick cooking spray.
2. Core the apples and cut a thin slice off the bottom of each apple so they can stand upright.
3. In a small bowl, mix together the chopped walnuts, honey or maple syrup, cinnamon, and nutmeg.
4. Stuff each apple with the walnut mixture, pressing down gently.
5. Place the stuffed apples in the prepared baking dish.
6. Pour the water into the bottom of the baking dish.
7. Bake for 25-30 minutes, or until the apples are tender and lightly browned.
8. Remove from the oven and let cool slightly before serving.
9. Enjoy these warm and comforting baked apples as a wholesome and satisfying dessert!

Nutrition Facts (per serving):

- Calories: 200
- Protein: 2g
- Fat: 5g
- Carbohydrates: 40g
- Fiber: 6g

Frozen Berry Yogurt Bark

Prep Time: 10 mins

Total Time: 3 hrs 10 mins

Servings: 4

Ingredients:

- 1 cup plain Greek yogurt
- 1 tablespoon honey or maple syrup
- 1/2 teaspoon vanilla extract
- 1 cup mixed berries (such as strawberries, blueberries, raspberries)
- 2 tablespoons chopped nuts (such as almonds, walnuts)

Directions:

1. In a mixing bowl, combine the plain Greek yogurt, honey or maple syrup, and vanilla extract. Stir until well combined.
2. Line a baking sheet with parchment paper.
3. Spread the yogurt mixture evenly onto the parchment paper, creating a thin layer.
4. Sprinkle the mixed berries and chopped nuts evenly over the yogurt layer, pressing them gently into the yogurt.
5. Place the baking sheet in the freezer and freeze for at least 3 hours, or until the yogurt bark is completely frozen.
6. Once frozen, remove the baking sheet from the freezer and break the yogurt bark into pieces.
7. Serve immediately and enjoy this refreshing and nutritious frozen berry yogurt bark as a guilt-free dessert or snack!

Nutrition Facts (per serving):

- Calories: 120

- Protein: 6g
- Fat: 5g
- Carbohydrates: 15g
- Fiber: 3g

Chia Seed Pudding with Berries

Prep Time: 5 mins

Total Time: 2 hrs 5 mins

Servings: 2

Ingredients:
- 1/4 cup chia seeds
- 1 cup coconut milk
- 1 tablespoon honey or maple syrup
- 1/2 teaspoon vanilla extract
- 1/2 cup mixed berries (such as strawberries, blueberries, raspberries)
- 2 tablespoons sliced almonds

Directions:
1. In a mixing bowl, combine the chia seeds, coconut milk, honey or maple syrup, and vanilla extract. Stir until well combined.
2. Cover and refrigerate for at least 2 hours, or overnight, to allow the chia pudding to thicken.
3. Once thickened, stir the chia pudding to evenly distribute the seeds.
4. Divide the chia pudding into serving bowls.
5. Top with mixed berries and sliced almonds.

6. Serve chilled and enjoy this creamy and nutritious chia seed pudding as a delightful dessert or snack!

Nutrition Facts (per serving):
- Calories: 220
- Protein: 5g
- Fat: 15g
- Carbohydrates: 20g
- Fiber: 8g

Baked Apple Chips

Prep Time: 10 mins

Total Time: 2 hrs 20 mins

Servings: 2

Ingredients:
- 2 apples (such as Granny Smith or Honey crisp)
- 1 tablespoon honey or maple syrup
- 1/2 teaspoon ground cinnamon

Directions:
1. Preheat the oven to 200°F (95°C). Line a baking sheet with parchment paper.
2. Core the apples and thinly slice them using a mandolin or sharp knife.
3. In a small bowl, whisk together the honey or maple syrup and ground cinnamon.
4. Arrange the apple slices in a single layer on the prepared baking sheet.
5. Brush the apple slices with the honey or maple syrup mixture.

6. Bake for 2 hours, flipping the apple slices halfway through, or until they are crispy and golden brown.
7. Remove from the oven and let cool completely before serving.
8. Enjoy these crunchy and naturally sweet baked apple chips as a healthy dessert or snack option!

Nutrition Facts (per serving):
- Calories: 120
- Protein: 1g
- Fat: 0g
- Carbohydrates: 30g
- Fiber: 5g

Coconut Banana Ice Cream

Prep Time: 5 mins

Total Time: 4 hrs 5 mins

Servings: 2

Ingredients:
- 2 ripe bananas, sliced and frozen
- 1/4 cup coconut milk
- 2 tablespoons shredded coconut
- 1 tablespoon honey or maple syrup (optional)

Directions:
1. Place the frozen banana slices, coconut milk, shredded coconut, and honey or maple syrup (if using) in a blender or food processor.
2. Blend until smooth and creamy, scraping down the sides as needed.

3. Transfer the mixture to a freezer-safe container and freeze for at least 4 hours, or until firm.
4. Once frozen, scoop the coconut banana ice cream into serving bowls.
5. Serve immediately and enjoy this creamy and naturally sweet ice cream as a refreshing dessert!

Nutrition Facts (per serving):
- Calories: 150
- Protein: 2g
- Fat: 5g
- Carbohydrates: 30g
- Fiber: 4g

Chocolate Avocado Mousse

Prep Time: 10 mins

Total Time: 10 mins

Servings: 2

Ingredients:
- 1 ripe avocado
- 2 tablespoons cocoa powder
- 2 tablespoons honey or maple syrup
- 1/2 teaspoon vanilla extract
- Pinch of salt

Directions:
1. Scoop the flesh of the ripe avocado into a blender or food processor.

2. Add the cocoa powder, honey or maple syrup, vanilla extract, and a pinch of salt.
3. Blend until smooth and creamy, scraping down the sides as needed.
4. Divide the chocolate avocado mousse into serving glasses.
5. Serve immediately and enjoy this rich and indulgent chocolate mousse as a guilt-free dessert option!

Nutrition Facts (per serving):
- Calories: 200
- Protein: 3g
- Fat: 12g
- Carbohydrates: 20g
- Fiber: 7g

Cinnamon Baked Pears

Prep Time: 10 mins

Total Time: 30 mins

Servings: 2

Ingredients:
- 2 ripe pears, halved and cored
- 1 tablespoon honey or maple syrup
- 1/2 teaspoon ground cinnamon
- 2 tablespoons chopped walnuts or pecans

Directions:
1. Preheat the oven to 375°F (190°C). Grease a baking dish with non-stick cooking spray.
2. Place the pear halves, cut side up, in the prepared baking dish.

3. Drizzle the honey or maple syrup over the pear halves.
4. Sprinkle ground cinnamon evenly over the pear halves.
5. Top each pear half with chopped walnuts or pecans.
6. Bake for 20-25 minutes, or until the pears are tender and golden brown.
7. Remove from the oven and let cool slightly before serving.
8. Enjoy these warm and fragrant cinnamon baked pears as a comforting and wholesome dessert!

Nutrition Facts (per serving):
- Calories: 160
- Protein: 2g
- Fat: 5g
- Carbohydrates: 30g
- Fiber: 6g

Coconut Chia Pudding with Fresh Fruit

Prep Time: 5 mins

Total Time: 2 hrs 5 mins

Servings: 2

Ingredients:
- 1/4 cup chia seeds
- 1 cup coconut milk
- 1 tablespoon honey or maple syrup
- 1/2 teaspoon vanilla extract
- 1/2 cup mixed fresh fruit (such as berries, mango, kiwi)
- 2 tablespoons unsweetened shredded coconut

Directions:

1. In a mixing bowl, combine the chia seeds, coconut milk, honey or maple syrup, and vanilla extract. Stir until well combined.
2. Cover and refrigerate for at least 2 hours, or overnight, to allow the chia pudding to thicken.
3. Once thickened, stir the chia pudding to evenly distribute the seeds.
4. Divide the chia pudding into serving bowls.
5. Top with mixed fresh fruit and shredded coconut.
6. Serve chilled and enjoy this creamy and nutritious coconut chia pudding as a delightful dessert or snack!

Nutrition Facts (per serving):
- Calories: 220
- Protein: 5g
- Fat: 15g
- Carbohydrates: 20g
- Fiber: 8g

Almond Flour Banana Bread

Prep Time: 15 mins

Total Time: 1 hr 15 mins

Servings: 8

Ingredients:
- 2 ripe bananas, mashed
- 2 eggs
- 1/4 cup honey or maple syrup
- 1/4 cup coconut oil, melted
- 1 teaspoon vanilla extract

- 2 cups almond flour
- 1 teaspoon baking powder
- 1/2 teaspoon ground cinnamon
- Pinch of salt
- Optional add-ins: chopped nuts, dried fruit

Directions:

1. Preheat the oven to 350°F (175°C). Grease a loaf pan with coconut oil or line with parchment paper.
2. In a large mixing bowl, combine the mashed bananas, eggs, honey or maple syrup, melted coconut oil, and vanilla extract. Mix until well combined.
3. Add the almond flour, baking powder, ground cinnamon, and salt to the wet ingredients. Stir until just combined.
4. If desired, fold in chopped nuts or dried fruit.
5. Pour the batter into the prepared loaf pan and spread it out evenly.
6. Bake for 50-60 minutes, or until a toothpick inserted into the center comes out clean.
7. Remove from the oven and let cool in the pan for 10 minutes before transferring to a wire rack to cool completely.
8. Slice and enjoy this delicious almond flour banana bread as a satisfying and wholesome dessert or snack!

Nutrition Facts (per serving):

- Calories: 250
- Protein: 7g
- Fat: 18g

- Carbohydrates: 20g
- Fiber: 4g

Baked Coconut Mango Oatmeal Cups

Prep Time: 10 mins

Total Time: 30 mins

Servings: 6

Ingredients:

- 1 cup rolled oats
- 1/4 cup unsweetened shredded coconut
- 1 ripe banana, mashed
- 1/2 cup coconut milk
- 1/4 cup honey or maple syrup
- 1/2 teaspoon vanilla extract
- 1/2 cup diced mango
- 2 tablespoons chopped nuts (such as almonds or walnuts)

Directions:

1. Preheat the oven to 350°F (175°C). Grease a muffin tin with coconut oil or line with silicone baking cups.
2. In a mixing bowl, combine the rolled oats, shredded coconut, mashed banana, coconut milk, honey or maple syrup, and vanilla extract. Mix until well combined.
3. Fold in the diced mango and chopped nuts.
4. Divide the oatmeal mixture evenly among the muffin cups.
5. Bake for 20-25 minutes, or until the oatmeal cups are set and lightly golden brown.

6. Remove from the oven and let cool in the muffin tin for 5 minutes before transferring to a wire rack to cool completely.
7. Serve these baked coconut mango oatmeal cups warm or at room temperature as a delicious and nutritious dessert or snack!

Nutrition Facts (per serving):
- Calories: 180
- Protein: 4g
- Fat: 7g
- Carbohydrates: 26g
- Fiber: 3g

Chocolate Peanut Butter Protein Balls

Prep Time: 15 mins

Total Time: 1 hr. 15 mins

Servings: 12

Ingredients:
- 1 cup rolled oats
- 1/2 cup natural peanut butter
- 1/4 cup honey or maple syrup
- 2 tablespoons cocoa powder
- 1/4 cup chocolate protein powder
- 1/4 cup unsweetened shredded coconut (optional)
- 2 tablespoons mini chocolate chips (optional)

Directions:
1. In a mixing bowl, combine the rolled oats, peanut butter, honey or maple syrup, cocoa powder, chocolate protein powder,

shredded coconut (if using), and mini chocolate chips (if using). Mix until well combined.
2. If the mixture is too dry, add a little more peanut butter or honey/maple syrup. If it's too wet, add more rolled oats.
3. Roll the mixture into bite-sized balls using your hands.
4. Place the protein balls on a baking sheet lined with parchment paper.
5. Refrigerate for at least 1 hour, or until firm.
6. Once firm, transfer the protein balls to an airtight container and store in the refrigerator until ready to eat.
7. Enjoy these chocolate peanut butter protein balls as a delicious and protein-rich dessert or snack!

Nutrition Facts (per serving - 1 ball):
- Calories: 130
- Protein: 5g
- Fat: 7g
- Carbohydrates: 13g
- Fiber: 2g

Apple Cinnamon Quinoa Breakfast Bars

Prep Time: 15 mins

Total Time: 40 mins

Servings: 9 bars

Ingredients:
- 1 cup cooked quinoa
- 1 large apple, peeled and grated
- 1/4 cup almond butter

- 1/4 cup honey or maple syrup
- 1 teaspoon ground cinnamon
- 1/4 teaspoon ground nutmeg
- 1/4 teaspoon salt
- 1/4 cup chopped nuts (such as walnuts or pecans)
- 1/4 cup dried cranberries or raisins

Directions:
1. Preheat the oven to 350°F (175°C). Grease a square baking dish or line it with parchment paper.
2. In a large mixing bowl, combine the cooked quinoa, grated apple, almond butter, honey or maple syrup, ground cinnamon, ground nutmeg, and salt. Mix until well combined.
3. Fold in the chopped nuts and dried cranberries or raisins.
4. Transfer the mixture to the prepared baking dish and press it down evenly with a spatula.
5. Bake for 25-30 minutes, or until the edges are golden brown and the bars are set.
6. Remove from the oven and let cool completely in the baking dish before slicing into bars.
7. Enjoy these apple cinnamon quinoa breakfast bars as a nutritious and satisfying dessert or snack option!

Nutrition Facts (per serving):
- Calories: 160
- Protein: 4g
- Fat: 7g
- Carbohydrates: 22g

- Fiber: 3g

Berry Avocado Parfait

Prep Time: 10 mins

Total Time: 10 mins

Servings: 2

Ingredients:

- 1 ripe avocado
- 1 cup mixed berries (such as strawberries, blueberries, raspberries)
- 1/4 cup unsweetened Greek yogurt or dairy-free yogurt alternative
- 2 tablespoons honey or maple syrup
- 1/4 cup granola
- Fresh mint leaves for garnish (optional)

Directions:

1. Scoop the flesh of the ripe avocado into a blender or food processor.
2. Add the mixed berries, Greek yogurt or dairy-free yogurt alternative, and honey or maple syrup to the blender.
3. Blend until smooth and creamy, scraping down the sides as needed.
4. Divide the berry avocado mixture into serving glasses.
5. Top each glass with a layer of granola.
6. Garnish with fresh mint leaves, if desired.
7. Serve immediately and enjoy this refreshing and nutritious berry avocado parfait as a delightful dessert or snack!

Nutrition Facts (per serving):

- Calories: 250
- Protein: 6g
- Fat: 12g
- Carbohydrates: 32g
- Fiber: 7g

Pumpkin Spice Chia Seed Pudding

Prep Time: 5 mins

Total Time: 2 hrs 5 mins

Servings: 2

Ingredients:

- 1/4 cup chia seeds
- 1 cup unsweetened almond milk or coconut milk
- 1/4 cup pumpkin puree
- 2 tablespoons honey or maple syrup
- 1/2 teaspoon vanilla extract
- 1/2 teaspoon ground cinnamon
- 1/4 teaspoon ground ginger
- Pinch of ground nutmeg
- Pinch of ground cloves
- 2 tablespoons chopped pecans or walnuts (optional)
- Whipped coconut cream for topping (optional)

Directions:

1. In a mixing bowl, combine the chia seeds, almond milk or coconut milk, pumpkin puree, honey or maple syrup, vanilla

extract, ground cinnamon, ground ginger, ground nutmeg, and ground cloves. Stir until well combined.
2. Cover and refrigerate for at least 2 hours, or overnight, to allow the chia pudding to thicken.
3. Once thickened, stir the chia pudding to evenly distribute the seeds.
4. Divide the pumpkin spice chia seed pudding into serving bowls.
5. Top with chopped pecans or walnuts and whipped coconut cream, if desired.
6. Serve chilled and enjoy this creamy and flavorful pumpkin spice chia seed pudding as a delicious dessert or snack!

Nutrition Facts (per serving):
- Calories: 220
- Protein: 6g
- Fat: 12g
- Carbohydrates: 25g
- Fiber: 9g

Coconut Mango Rice Pudding

Prep Time: 10 mins

Total Time: 40 mins

Servings: 4

Ingredients:
- 1/2 cup Arborio rice
- 1 can (13.5 oz) coconut milk
- 1 cup water
- 2 tablespoons honey or maple syrup

- 1/2 teaspoon vanilla extract
- 1 ripe mango, diced
- Unsweetened shredded coconut for garnish (optional)

Directions:
1. In a saucepan, combine the Arborio rice, coconut milk, water, honey or maple syrup, and vanilla extract. Stir well.
2. Bring the mixture to a boil over medium heat.
3. Reduce the heat to low, cover, and simmer for 25-30 minutes, stirring occasionally, until the rice is tender and the mixture has thickened.
4. Remove from heat and let cool slightly.
5. Divide the coconut mango rice pudding into serving bowls.
6. Top with diced mango and shredded coconut, if desired.
7. Serve warm or chilled and enjoy this creamy and tropical coconut mango rice pudding as a delightful dessert!

Nutrition Facts (per serving):
- Calories: 290
- Protein: 4g
- Fat: 18g
- Carbohydrates: 31g
- Fiber: 2g

Dark Chocolate Avocado Mousse

Prep Time: 10 mins

Total Time: 10 mins

Servings: 2

Ingredients:

- 1 ripe avocado
- 2 tablespoons cocoa powder
- 2 tablespoons honey or maple syrup
- 1/2 teaspoon vanilla extract
- Pinch of salt
- Dark chocolate shavings for garnish (optional)

Directions:

1. Scoop the flesh of the ripe avocado into a blender or food processor.
2. Add the cocoa powder, honey or maple syrup, vanilla extract, and a pinch of salt to the blender.
3. Blend until smooth and creamy, scraping down the sides as needed.
4. Divide the dark chocolate avocado mousse into serving glasses.
5. Garnish with dark chocolate shavings, if desired.
6. Serve immediately and enjoy this rich and decadent dark chocolate avocado mousse as a guilt-free dessert or snack!

Nutrition Facts (per serving):

- Calories: 200
- Protein: 3g
- Fat: 14g
- Carbohydrates: 20g
- Fiber: 7g

Banana Oatmeal Cookies

Prep Time: 10 mins

Total Time: 20 mins

Servings: 12 cookies

Ingredients:

- 2 ripe bananas, mashed
- 1 cup rolled oats
- 1/4 cup almond flour
- 2 tablespoons honey or maple syrup
- 1/4 teaspoon ground cinnamon
- 1/4 teaspoon vanilla extract
- Pinch of salt
- 2 tablespoons dark chocolate chips (optional)
- 2 tablespoons chopped nuts (such as walnuts or almonds) (optional)

Directions:

1. Preheat the oven to 350°F (175°C). Line a baking sheet with parchment paper.
2. In a mixing bowl, combine the mashed bananas, rolled oats, almond flour, honey or maple syrup, ground cinnamon, vanilla extract, and a pinch of salt. Mix until well combined.
3. If desired, fold in dark chocolate chips and chopped nuts.
4. Drop spoonfuls of the cookie dough onto the prepared baking sheet, spacing them apart.
5. Flatten each cookie slightly with the back of a spoon.
6. Bake for 10-12 minutes, or until the cookies are golden brown around the edges.

7. Remove from the oven and let cool on the baking sheet for 5 minutes before transferring to a wire rack to cool completely.
8. Enjoy these banana oatmeal cookies as a wholesome and satisfying dessert or snack option!

Nutrition Facts (per serving - 1 cookie):
- Calories: 80
- Protein: 2g
- Fat: 2g
- Carbohydrates: 15g
- Fiber: 2g

SOUP RECIPES

Creamy Butternut Squash Soup

Prep Time: 15 mins

Total Time: 40 mins

Servings: 4

Ingredients:

- 1 medium butternut squash, peeled, seeded, and cubed
- 1 onion, chopped
- 2 cloves garlic, minced
- 4 cups vegetable broth
- 1/2 teaspoon ground cinnamon
- 1/4 teaspoon ground nutmeg
- Salt and pepper to taste
- 1/2 cup coconut milk or almond milk
- Fresh parsley or chives for garnish (optional)

Directions:

1. In a large pot, heat some olive oil over medium heat. Add the chopped onion and minced garlic, and sauté until softened, about 5 minutes.
2. Add the cubed butternut squash to the pot, along with the vegetable broth, ground cinnamon, ground nutmeg, salt, and pepper. Bring to a boil.
3. Reduce the heat to low, cover, and simmer for 20-25 minutes, or until the squash is tender.

4. Use an immersion blender to blend the soup until smooth. Alternatively, transfer the soup to a blender and blend in batches until smooth.
5. Stir in the coconut milk or almond milk until well combined.
6. Taste and adjust seasoning if needed.
7. Ladle the soup into bowls and garnish with fresh parsley or chives, if desired.
8. Serve hot and enjoy this creamy and comforting butternut squash soup!

Nutrition Facts (per serving):
- Calories: 120
- Protein: 2g
- Fat: 3g
- Carbohydrates: 24g
- Fiber: 5g

Lentil and Vegetable Soup

Prep Time: 15 mins

Total Time: 45 mins

Servings: 6

Ingredients:
- 1 cup dried green lentils, rinsed and drained
- 1 onion, chopped
- 2 carrots, diced
- 2 celery stalks, diced
- 2 cloves garlic, minced
- 4 cups vegetable broth

- 1 can (14 oz) diced tomatoes
- 1 teaspoon ground cumin
- 1 teaspoon ground coriander
- 1/2 teaspoon smoked paprika
- Salt and pepper to taste
- Fresh parsley or cilantro for garnish (optional)

Directions:
1. In a large pot, heat some olive oil over medium heat. Add the chopped onion, diced carrots, diced celery, and minced garlic, and sauté until softened, about 5 minutes.
2. Add the rinsed lentils, vegetable broth, diced tomatoes (with their juices), ground cumin, ground coriander, smoked paprika, salt, and pepper to the pot. Stir to combine.
3. Bring the soup to a boil, then reduce the heat to low, cover, and simmer for 25-30 minutes, or until the lentils are tender.
4. Taste and adjust seasoning if needed.
5. Ladle the soup into bowls and garnish with fresh parsley or cilantro, if desired.
6. Serve hot and enjoy this hearty and nutritious lentil and vegetable soup!

Nutrition Facts (per serving):
- Calories: 180
- Protein: 10g
- Fat: 1g
- Carbohydrates: 32g
- Fiber: 12g

Roasted Tomato Basil Soup

Prep Time: 10 mins

Total Time: 50 mins

Servings: 4

Ingredients:

- 2 lbs ripe tomatoes, halved
- 1 onion, chopped
- 3 cloves garlic, minced
- 2 tablespoons olive oil
- 4 cups vegetable broth
- 1/4 cup fresh basil leaves, chopped
- Salt and pepper to taste
- Balsamic glaze for garnish (optional)

Directions:

1. Preheat the oven to 400°F (200°C). Place the halved tomatoes on a baking sheet, cut side up. Drizzle with olive oil and season with salt and pepper.
2. Roast the tomatoes in the preheated oven for 30-35 minutes, or until softened and slightly caramelized.
3. In a large pot, heat some olive oil over medium heat. Add the chopped onion and minced garlic, and sauté until softened, about 5 minutes.
4. Add the roasted tomatoes (including any juices) to the pot, along with the vegetable broth and chopped basil. Bring to a boil.

5. Reduce the heat to low, cover, and simmer for 10-15 minutes to allow the flavors to meld together.
6. Use an immersion blender to blend the soup until smooth. Alternatively, transfer the soup to a blender and blend in batches until smooth.
7. Taste and adjust seasoning if needed.
8. Ladle the soup into bowls and drizzle with balsamic glaze, if desired.
9. Serve hot and enjoy this rich and flavorful roasted tomato basil soup!

Nutrition Facts (per serving):
- Calories: 150
- Protein: 3g
- Fat: 7g
- Carbohydrates: 20g
- Fiber: 5g

Ginger Carrot Soup

Prep Time: 10 mins

Total Time: 35 mins

Servings: 4

Ingredients:
- 1 lb carrots, peeled and chopped
- 1 onion, chopped
- 2 cloves garlic, minced
- 2 tablespoons fresh ginger, grated
- 4 cups vegetable broth

- 1/2 cup coconut milk or almond milk
- 1 tablespoon olive oil
- Salt and pepper to taste
- Fresh cilantro for garnish (optional)

Directions:

1. In a large pot, heat some olive oil over medium heat. Add the chopped onion, minced garlic, and grated ginger, and sauté until fragrant, about 2 minutes.
2. Add the chopped carrots to the pot and sauté for another 5 minutes.
3. Pour in the vegetable broth and bring to a boil. Reduce the heat to low, cover, and simmer for 20-25 minutes, or until the carrots are tender.
4. Use an immersion blender to blend the soup until smooth. Alternatively, transfer the soup to a blender and blend in batches until smooth.
5. Stir in the coconut milk or almond milk until well combined.
6. Taste and adjust seasoning if needed.
7. Ladle the soup into bowls and garnish with fresh cilantro, if desired.
8. Serve hot and enjoy this warming and comforting ginger carrot soup!

Nutrition Facts (per serving):

- Calories: 120
- Protein: 2g
- Fat: 5g

- Carbohydrates: 18g
- Fiber: 5g

Creamy Mushroom Soup

Prep Time: 10 mins

Total Time: 30 mins

Servings: 4

Ingredients:

- 1 lb mushrooms, sliced (button mushrooms or cremini mushrooms)
- 1 onion, chopped
- 2 cloves garlic, minced
- 4 cups vegetable broth
- 1/2 cup coconut milk or almond milk
- 2 tablespoons olive oil
- 2 tablespoons all-purpose flour or gluten-free flour
- Salt and pepper to taste
- Fresh thyme for garnish (optional)

Directions:

1. In a large pot, heat some olive oil over medium heat. Add the chopped onion and minced garlic, and sauté until softened, about 5 minutes.
2. Add the sliced mushrooms to the pot and sauté until they release their moisture and start to brown, about 8-10 minutes.
3. Sprinkle the flour over the mushrooms and stir to coat.
4. Pour in the vegetable broth and bring to a boil. Reduce the heat to low, cover, and simmer for 10-15 minutes.

5. Use an immersion blender to blend the soup until smooth. Alternatively, transfer the soup to a blender and blend in batches until smooth.
6. Stir in the coconut milk or almond milk until well combined.
7. Taste and adjust seasoning if needed.
8. Ladle the soup into bowls and garnish with fresh thyme, if desired.
9. Serve hot and enjoy this creamy and flavorful mushroom soup!

Nutrition Facts (per serving):
- Calories: 140
- Protein: 4g
- Fat: 8g
- Carbohydrates: 14g
- Fiber: 3g

Spicy Black Bean Soup

Prep Time: 10 mins

Total Time: 30 mins

Servings: 4

Ingredients:
- 2 cans (15 oz each) black beans, drained and rinsed
- 1 onion, chopped
- 2 cloves garlic, minced
- 1 bell pepper, diced
- 1 jalapeño pepper, diced (seeds removed for less heat)
- 4 cups vegetable broth
- 1 teaspoon ground cumin

- 1 teaspoon chili powder
- 1/2 teaspoon smoked paprika
- Salt and pepper to taste
- Juice of 1 lime
- Fresh cilantro for garnish (optional)
- Avocado slices for garnish (optional)
- Tortilla chips or strips for serving (optional)

Directions:

1. In a large pot, heat some olive oil over medium heat. Add the chopped onion, minced garlic, diced bell pepper, and diced jalapeño pepper, and sauté until softened, about 5 minutes.
2. Add the drained and rinsed black beans to the pot, along with the vegetable broth, ground cumin, chili powder, smoked paprika, salt, and pepper. Stir to combine.
3. Bring the soup to a boil, then reduce the heat to low, cover, and simmer for 15-20 minutes to allow the flavors to meld together.
4. Use an immersion blender to blend a portion of the soup until smooth, leaving some chunks of beans and vegetables for texture. Alternatively, transfer a portion of the soup to a blender and blend until smooth, then return it to the pot.
5. Stir in the lime juice until well combined.
6. Taste and adjust seasoning if needed.
7. Ladle the soup into bowls and garnish with fresh cilantro, avocado slices, and tortilla chips or strips, if desired.
8. Serve hot and enjoy this hearty and flavorful spicy black bean soup!

Nutrition Facts (per serving):
- Calories: 220
- Protein: 10g
- Fat: 2g
- Carbohydrates: 40g
- Fiber: 12g

Butternut Squash Soup

Prep Time: 15 mins

Total Time: 45 mins

Servings: 4

Ingredients:
- 1 medium butternut squash, peeled, seeded, and diced
- 1 onion, chopped
- 2 cloves garlic, minced
- 1 carrot, peeled and chopped
- 4 cups vegetable broth
- 1 teaspoon dried thyme
- 1/2 teaspoon ground cinnamon
- Salt and pepper to taste
- 2 tablespoons olive oil
- Fresh parsley for garnish (optional)
- Pumpkin seeds for garnish (optional)

Directions:
1. Heat olive oil in a large pot over medium heat. Add the chopped onion, minced garlic, and chopped carrot. Sauté until softened, about 5 minutes.

2. Add the diced butternut squash to the pot along with the vegetable broth, dried thyme, ground cinnamon, salt, and pepper. Bring to a boil, then reduce heat to low, cover, and simmer for 25-30 minutes until the squash is tender.
3. Use an immersion blender to blend the soup until smooth. Alternatively, transfer the soup to a blender and blend in batches until smooth.
4. Taste and adjust seasoning if needed.
5. Ladle the soup into bowls and garnish with fresh parsley and pumpkin seeds, if desired.
6. Serve hot and enjoy this creamy and comforting butternut squash soup!

Nutrition Facts (per serving):
- Calories: 180
- Protein: 3g
- Fat: 7g
- Carbohydrates: 30g
- Fiber: 6g

Lentil Soup

Prep Time: 10 mins

Total Time: 40 mins

Servings: 4

Ingredients:
- 1 cup dried green or brown lentils, rinsed
- 1 onion, chopped
- 2 cloves garlic, minced

- 1 carrot, peeled and chopped
- 1 stalk celery, chopped
- 4 cups vegetable broth
- 1 can (14 oz) diced tomatoes
- 1 teaspoon ground cumin
- 1 teaspoon paprika
- Salt and pepper to taste
- Fresh parsley for garnish (optional)
- Lemon wedges for serving (optional)

Directions:

1. In a large pot, heat some olive oil over medium heat. Add the chopped onion, minced garlic, chopped carrot, and chopped celery. Sauté until softened, about 5 minutes.
2. Add the rinsed lentils, vegetable broth, diced tomatoes, ground cumin, paprika, salt, and pepper to the pot. Bring to a boil, then reduce heat to low, cover, and simmer for 25-30 minutes until the lentils are tender.
3. Taste and adjust seasoning if needed.
4. Ladle the soup into bowls and garnish with fresh parsley. Serve with lemon wedges on the side for a burst of freshness, if desired.
5. Serve hot and enjoy this hearty and nutritious lentil soup!

Nutrition Facts (per serving):

- Calories: 220
- Protein: 12g
- Fat: 1g

- Carbohydrates: 40g
- Fiber: 15g

Tomato Basil Soup

Prep Time: 10 mins

Total Time: 35 mins

Servings: 4

Ingredients:

- 1 tablespoon olive oil
- 1 onion, chopped
- 2 cloves garlic, minced
- 2 cans (14 oz each) diced tomatoes
- 2 cups vegetable broth
- 1 teaspoon dried basil
- 1/2 teaspoon dried oregano
- Salt and pepper to taste
- 1/4 cup coconut milk or almond milk (optional, for creaminess)
- Fresh basil leaves for garnish (optional)
- Croutons for serving (optional)

Directions:

1. Heat olive oil in a large pot over medium heat. Add the chopped onion and minced garlic, and sauté until softened, about 5 minutes.
2. Add the diced tomatoes (with their juices), vegetable broth, dried basil, dried oregano, salt, and pepper to the pot. Bring to a boil, then reduce heat to low, cover, and simmer for 20-25 minutes.

3. Use an immersion blender to blend the soup until smooth. Alternatively, transfer the soup to a blender and blend in batches until smooth.
4. Stir in the coconut milk or almond milk if using, until well combined.
5. Taste and adjust seasoning if needed.
6. Ladle the soup into bowls and garnish with fresh basil leaves and croutons, if desired.
7. Serve hot and enjoy this classic and comforting tomato basil soup!

Nutrition Facts (per serving):
- Calories: 120
- Protein: 3g
- Fat: 3g
- Carbohydrates: 20g
- Fiber: 5g

Carrot Ginger Soup

Prep Time: 10 mins

Total Time: 35 mins

Servings: 4

Ingredients:
- 1 tablespoon olive oil
- 1 onion, chopped
- 2 cloves garlic, minced
- 1 tablespoon fresh ginger, minced
- 4 cups chopped carrots

- 4 cups vegetable broth
- 1/2 teaspoon ground turmeric
- Salt and pepper to taste
- Coconut cream or yogurt for serving (optional)
- Fresh cilantro for garnish (optional)

Directions:

1. In a large pot, heat olive oil over medium heat. Add the chopped onion, minced garlic, and minced ginger, and sauté until fragrant, about 2 minutes.
2. Add the chopped carrots to the pot and sauté for another 5 minutes.
3. Pour in the vegetable broth, ground turmeric, salt, and pepper. Bring to a boil, then reduce heat to low, cover, and simmer for 20-25 minutes until the carrots are tender.
4. Use an immersion blender to blend the soup until smooth. Alternatively, transfer the soup to a blender and blend in batches until smooth.
5. Taste and adjust seasoning if needed.
6. Ladle the soup into bowls and drizzle with coconut cream or yogurt, if using. Garnish with fresh cilantro, if desired.
7. Serve hot and enjoy this vibrant and flavorful carrot ginger soup!

Nutrition Facts (per serving):

- Calories: 110
- Protein: 2g
- Fat: 4g

- Carbohydrates: 18g
- Fiber: 5g

Spinach and Potato Soup

Prep Time: 15 mins

Total Time: 40 mins

Servings: 4

Ingredients:

- 1 tablespoon olive oil
- 1 onion, chopped
- 2 cloves garlic, minced
- 2 large potatoes, peeled and diced
- 4 cups vegetable broth
- 4 cups fresh spinach leaves
- 1/2 teaspoon dried thyme
- Salt and pepper to taste
- Lemon wedges for serving (optional)

Directions:

1. Heat olive oil in a large pot over medium heat. Add the chopped onion and minced garlic, and sauté until softened, about 5 minutes.
2. Add the diced potatoes to the pot and sauté for another 5 minutes.
3. Pour in the vegetable broth and bring to a boil. Reduce heat to low, cover, and simmer for 15-20 minutes until the potatoes are tender.

4. Stir in the fresh spinach leaves and dried thyme. Cook for an additional 5 minutes until the spinach is wilted.
5. Use an immersion blender to blend a portion of the soup until smooth, leaving some chunks of potatoes and spinach for texture. Alternatively, transfer a portion of the soup to a blender and blend until smooth, then return it to the pot.
6. Taste and adjust seasoning if needed.
7. Ladle the soup into bowls and serve with lemon wedges on the side for a fresh squeeze of flavor, if desired.
8. Serve hot and enjoy this nutritious and comforting spinach and potato soup!

Nutrition Facts (per serving):
- Calories: 160
- Protein: 4g
- Fat: 3g
- Carbohydrates: 30g
- Fiber: 5g

Vegetable Quinoa Soup

Prep Time: 10 mins

Total Time: 35 mins

Servings: 4

Ingredients:
- 1 tablespoon olive oil
- 1 onion, diced
- 2 cloves garlic, minced
- 2 carrots, peeled and diced

- 2 celery stalks, diced
- 1 bell pepper, diced
- 1 cup quinoa, rinsed
- 6 cups vegetable broth
- 1 teaspoon dried thyme
- Salt and pepper to taste
- Fresh parsley for garnish (optional)

Directions:

1. In a large pot, heat olive oil over medium heat. Add the diced onion and minced garlic, and sauté until softened, about 5 minutes.
2. Add the diced carrots, celery, and bell pepper to the pot. Cook for another 5 minutes until the vegetables are slightly softened.
3. Stir in the rinsed quinoa, vegetable broth, dried thyme, salt, and pepper. Bring to a boil, then reduce heat to low, cover, and simmer for 20 minutes until the quinoa is cooked and the vegetables are tender.
4. Taste and adjust seasoning if needed.
5. Ladle the soup into bowls and garnish with fresh parsley, if desired.
6. Serve hot and enjoy this hearty and nutritious vegetable quinoa soup!

Nutritional Information (per serving):

- Calories: 250
- Protein: 8g
- Fat: 5g

- Carbohydrates: 45g
- Fiber: 8g

Creamy Cauliflower Soup

Prep Time: 10 mins

Total Time: 35 mins

Servings: 4

Ingredients:

- 1 tablespoon olive oil
- 1 onion, chopped
- 2 cloves garlic, minced
- 1 head cauliflower, chopped into florets
- 4 cups vegetable broth
- 1/2 teaspoon dried thyme
- Salt and pepper to taste
- 1/2 cup coconut milk (from a can)
- Fresh chives for garnish (optional)

Directions:

1. Heat olive oil in a large pot over medium heat. Add the chopped onion and minced garlic, and sauté until softened, about 5 minutes.
2. Add the cauliflower florets to the pot along with the vegetable broth, dried thyme, salt, and pepper. Bring to a boil, then reduce heat to low, cover, and simmer for 20 minutes until the cauliflower is tender.

3. Use an immersion blender to blend the soup until smooth. Alternatively, transfer the soup to a blender and blend in batches until smooth.
4. Stir in the coconut milk until well combined and heated through.
5. Taste and adjust seasoning if needed.
6. Ladle the soup into bowls and garnish with fresh chives, if desired.
7. Serve hot and enjoy this creamy and delicious cauliflower soup!

Nutritional Information (per serving):
- Calories: 180
- Protein: 5g
- Fat: 10g
- Carbohydrates: 20g
- Fiber: 5g

Lentil and Vegetable Soup

Prep Time: 10 mins

Total Time: 45 mins

Servings: 4

Ingredients:
- 1 tablespoon olive oil
- 1 onion, diced
- 2 cloves garlic, minced
- 1 carrot, diced
- 1 celery stalk, diced
- 1 cup dried lentils, rinsed

- 4 cups vegetable broth
- 1 teaspoon ground cumin
- 1/2 teaspoon paprika
- Salt and pepper to taste
- Fresh parsley for garnish (optional)

Directions:

1. Heat olive oil in a large pot over medium heat. Add the diced onion and minced garlic, and sauté until softened, about 5 minutes.
2. Add the diced carrot and celery to the pot, and cook for another 5 minutes until slightly softened.
3. Stir in the rinsed lentils, vegetable broth, ground cumin, paprika, salt, and pepper. Bring to a boil, then reduce heat to low, cover, and simmer for 30 minutes until the lentils are tender.
4. Taste and adjust seasoning if needed.
5. Ladle the soup into bowls and garnish with fresh parsley, if desired.
6. Serve hot and enjoy this hearty and nutritious lentil and vegetable soup!

Nutritional Information (per serving):

- Calories: 220
- Protein: 12g
- Fat: 3g
- Carbohydrates: 35g
- Fiber: 12g

Butternut Squash Soup

Prep Time: 15 mins

Total Time: 40 mins

Servings: 4

Ingredients:

- 1 tablespoon olive oil
- 1 onion, chopped
- 2 cloves garlic, minced
- 1 medium butternut squash, peeled, seeded, and chopped
- 4 cups vegetable broth
- 1 teaspoon ground cinnamon
- 1/2 teaspoon ground nutmeg
- Salt and pepper to taste
- Coconut cream for serving (optional)
- Fresh thyme for garnish (optional)

Directions:

1. In a large pot, heat olive oil over medium heat. Add the chopped onion and minced garlic, and sauté until softened, about 5 minutes.
2. Add the chopped butternut squash to the pot along with the vegetable broth, ground cinnamon, ground nutmeg, salt, and pepper. Bring to a boil, then reduce heat to low, cover, and simmer for 20 minutes until the squash is tender.
3. Use an immersion blender to blend the soup until smooth. Alternatively, transfer the soup to a blender and blend in batches until smooth.

4. Taste and adjust seasoning if needed.
5. Ladle the soup into bowls and swirl in some coconut cream, if using. Garnish with fresh thyme, if desired.
6. Serve hot and enjoy this velvety and comforting butternut squash soup!

Nutritional Information (per serving):
- Calories: 180
- Protein: 3g
- Fat: 5g
- Carbohydrates: 35g
- Fiber: 6g

Tomato Basil Soup

Prep Time: 10 mins

Total Time: 30 mins

Servings: 4

Ingredients:
- 1 tablespoon olive oil
- 1 onion, chopped
- 2 cloves garlic, minced
- 2 cans (14 oz each) diced tomatoes
- 2 cups vegetable broth
- 1 teaspoon dried basil
- 1/2 teaspoon dried oregano
- Salt and pepper to taste
- Fresh basil leaves for garnish (optional)
- Croutons for serving (optional)

Directions:

1. Heat olive oil in a large pot over medium heat. Add the chopped onion and minced garlic, and sauté until softened, about 5 minutes.
2. Add the diced tomatoes (with their juices) to the pot along with the vegetable broth, dried basil, dried oregano, salt, and pepper. Bring to a boil, then reduce heat to low, cover, and simmer for 15 minutes.
3. Use an immersion blender to blend the soup until smooth. Alternatively, transfer the soup to a blender and blend in batches until smooth.
4. Taste and adjust seasoning if needed.
5. Ladle the soup into bowls and garnish with fresh basil leaves, if desired. Serve with croutons on the side for added texture, if desired.
6. Serve hot and enjoy this classic and comforting tomato basil soup!

Nutritional Information (per serving):

- Calories: 120
- Protein: 3g
- Fat: 3g
- Carbohydrates: 20g
- Fiber: 5g

Chicken and Vegetable Soup

Prep Time: 15 mins

Total Time: 45 mins

Servings: 4

Ingredients:

- 1 tablespoon olive oil
- 1 onion, diced
- 2 cloves garlic, minced
- 2 carrots, diced
- 2 celery stalks, diced
- 1 medium potato, diced
- 4 cups low-sodium chicken broth
- 2 cups shredded cooked chicken breast
- 1 teaspoon dried thyme
- Salt and pepper to taste
- Fresh parsley for garnish (optional)

Directions:

1. In a large pot, heat olive oil over medium heat. Add diced onion and minced garlic, and sauté until softened, about 5 minutes.
2. Add diced carrots, celery, and potato to the pot, and cook for another 5 minutes until slightly softened.
3. Pour in the chicken broth and bring to a boil. Reduce heat to low, cover, and simmer for 20 minutes until vegetables are tender.
4. Stir in shredded cooked chicken breast and dried thyme. Simmer for another 10 minutes.
5. Season with salt and pepper to taste.
6. Ladle the soup into bowls, garnish with fresh parsley if desired, and serve hot.

Nutritional Information (per serving):
- Calories: 210
- Protein: 20g
- Fat: 6g
- Carbohydrates: 18g
- Fiber: 3g

Lentil and Spinach Soup

Prep Time: 10 mins

Total Time: 40 mins

Servings: 4

Ingredients:
- 1 tablespoon olive oil
- 1 onion, chopped
- 2 cloves garlic, minced
- 1 carrot, diced
- 1 celery stalk, diced
- 1 cup dried green lentils, rinsed
- 4 cups vegetable broth
- 2 cups fresh spinach leaves
- 1 teaspoon ground cumin
- Salt and pepper to taste
- Lemon wedges for serving (optional)

Directions:
1. Heat olive oil in a large pot over medium heat. Add chopped onion and minced garlic, and sauté until softened, about 5 minutes.

2. Add diced carrot and celery to the pot, and cook for another 5 minutes until slightly softened.
3. Stir in rinsed lentils, vegetable broth, and ground cumin. Bring to a boil, then reduce heat to low, cover, and simmer for 25 minutes until lentils are tender.
4. Add fresh spinach leaves to the pot and stir until wilted, about 3 minutes.
5. Season with salt and pepper to taste.
6. Serve the soup hot with lemon wedges on the side for squeezing over the soup if desired.

Nutritional Information (per serving):
- Calories: 240
- Protein: 13g
- Fat: 3g
- Carbohydrates: 40g
- Fiber: 17g

Butternut Squash Soup

Prep Time: 15 mins

Total Time: 45 mins

Servings: 4

Ingredients:
- 1 tablespoon olive oil
- 1 onion, chopped
- 2 cloves garlic, minced
- 1 butternut squash, peeled, seeded, and diced
- 2 carrots, chopped

- 4 cups vegetable broth
- 1 teaspoon ground cinnamon
- 1/2 teaspoon ground nutmeg
- Salt and pepper to taste
- Plain yogurt or coconut cream for garnish (optional)
- Fresh chives for garnish (optional)

Directions:

1. In a large pot, heat olive oil over medium heat. Add chopped onion and minced garlic, and sauté until softened, about 5 minutes.
2. Add diced butternut squash and chopped carrots to the pot, and cook for another 5 minutes until slightly softened.
3. Pour in vegetable broth and add ground cinnamon and ground nutmeg. Bring to a boil, then reduce heat to low, cover, and simmer for 25 minutes until vegetables are tender.
4. Use an immersion blender to puree the soup until smooth. Alternatively, transfer the soup to a blender and blend in batches until smooth.
5. Season with salt and pepper to taste.
6. Ladle the soup into bowls, and garnish with a dollop of plain yogurt or coconut cream and fresh chives if desired.

Nutritional Information (per serving):

- Calories: 180
- Protein: 3g
- Fat: 4g
- Carbohydrates: 35g

- Fiber: 7g

Mushroom Barley Soup

Prep Time: 15 mins

Total Time: 1 hour

Servings: 4

Ingredients:

- 1 tablespoon olive oil
- 1 onion, chopped
- 2 cloves garlic, minced
- 8 oz mushrooms, sliced (such as cremini or button mushrooms)
- 1 carrot, diced
- 1 celery stalk, diced
- 1/2 cup pearl barley, rinsed
- 4 cups vegetable broth
- 1 teaspoon dried thyme
- Salt and pepper to taste
- Fresh parsley for garnish (optional)

Directions:

1. Heat olive oil in a large pot over medium heat. Add chopped onion and minced garlic, and sauté until softened, about 5 minutes.
2. Add sliced mushrooms, diced carrot, and diced celery to the pot, and cook for another 5 minutes until mushrooms release their juices.

3. Stir in rinsed pearl barley, vegetable broth, and dried thyme. Bring to a boil, then reduce heat to low, cover, and simmer for 40 minutes until barley is tender.
4. Season with salt and pepper to taste.
5. Ladle the soup into bowls, and garnish with fresh parsley if desired.

Nutritional Information (per serving):
- Calories: 220
- Protein: 7g
- Fat: 4g
- Carbohydrates: 40g
- Fiber: 8g

Tomato and White Bean Soup

Prep Time: 10 mins

Total Time: 30 mins

Servings: 4

Ingredients:
- 1 tablespoon olive oil
- 1 onion, chopped
- 2 cloves garlic, minced
- 1 can (15 oz) diced tomatoes
- 2 cups vegetable broth
- 1 can (15 oz) cannellini beans, drained and rinsed
- 1 teaspoon dried basil
- 1/2 teaspoon dried oregano
- Salt and pepper to taste

- Fresh basil leaves for garnish (optional)
- Grated Parmesan cheese for garnish (optional)

Directions:

1. In a large pot, heat olive oil over medium heat. Add chopped onion and minced garlic, and sauté until softened, about 5 minutes.
2. Add diced tomatoes (with their juices) to the pot, along with vegetable broth, cannellini beans, dried basil, and dried oregano. Bring to a boil, then reduce heat to low, cover, and simmer for 15 minutes.
3. Use an immersion blender to partially blend the soup, leaving some chunks of tomatoes and beans for texture. Alternatively, transfer a portion of the soup to a blender and blend until smooth, then return it to the pot.
4. Season with salt and pepper to taste.
5. Ladle the soup into bowls, and garnish with fresh basil leaves and grated Parmesan cheese if desired.

Nutritional Information (per serving):

- Calories: 180
- Protein: 8g
- Fat: 4g
- Carbohydrates: 30g
- Fiber: 7g

SNACKS RECIPES

Nutty Energy Bites

Prep Time: 15 mins

Total Time: 15 mins

Servings: 12 bites

Ingredients:
- 1 cup rolled oats
- 1/2 cup creamy almond butter
- 1/4 cup honey or maple syrup
- 1/4 cup chopped nuts (such as almonds, walnuts, or cashews)
- 1/4 cup dried fruit (such as raisins, cranberries, or apricots), chopped
- 1 tablespoon chia seeds
- 1/2 teaspoon vanilla extract
- Pinch of salt

Directions:
1. In a large mixing bowl, combine rolled oats, almond butter, honey or maple syrup, chopped nuts, dried fruit, chia seeds, vanilla extract, and a pinch of salt.
2. Stir until well combined and the mixture holds together.
3. Using your hands, roll the mixture into small balls, about 1 inch in diameter.
4. Place the energy bites on a baking sheet lined with parchment paper.
5. Refrigerate for at least 30 minutes to firm up.

6. Once firm, transfer the energy bites to an airtight container and store in the refrigerator for up to 1 week.
7. Enjoy these nutritious and satisfying energy bites as a quick and convenient snack!

Nutrition Facts (per serving - 1 bite):
- Calories: 120
- Protein: 3g
- Fat: 6g
- Carbohydrates: 14g
- Fiber: 2g

Avocado Toast with Tomato and Basil

Prep Time: 5 mins

Total Time: 10 mins

Servings: 2

Ingredients:
- 2 slices whole grain bread, toasted
- 1 ripe avocado, mashed
- 1 tomato, sliced
- Fresh basil leaves
- Salt and pepper to taste
- Optional toppings: red pepper flakes, balsamic glaze

Directions:
1. Spread the mashed avocado evenly onto the toasted whole grain bread slices.
2. Top each slice with tomato slices and fresh basil leaves.
3. Season with salt and pepper to taste.

4. For added flavor, sprinkle with red pepper flakes and drizzle with balsamic glaze, if desired.
5. Serve immediately and enjoy this simple and delicious avocado toast!

Nutrition Facts (per serving):
- Calories: 180
- Protein: 5g
- Fat: 10g
- Carbohydrates: 20g
- Fiber: 8g

Greek Yogurt Parfait

Prep Time: 5 mins

Total Time: 5 mins

Servings: 1

Ingredients:
- 1/2 cup plain Greek yogurt
- 1/4 cup granola
- 1/4 cup mixed berries (such as strawberries, blueberries, raspberries)
- 1 tablespoon honey or maple syrup (optional)

Directions:
1. In a serving glass or bowl, layer the plain Greek yogurt, granola, and mixed berries.
2. Drizzle with honey or maple syrup, if using.
3. Repeat the layers until the glass or bowl is full.

4. Serve immediately and enjoy this creamy and refreshing Greek yogurt parfait!

Nutrition Facts (per serving):
- Calories: 250
- Protein: 15g
- Fat: 6g
- Carbohydrates: 35g
- Fiber: 5g

Hummus and Veggie Stuffed Pita Pockets

Prep Time: 10 mins

Total Time: 10 mins

Servings: 2

Ingredients:
- 2 whole grain pita pockets
- 1/2 cup hummus
- 1/2 cucumber, thinly sliced
- 1/2 bell pepper, thinly sliced
- 1/4 cup shredded carrots
- Handful of spinach leaves

Directions:
1. Warm the whole grain pita pockets in the microwave or toaster oven until slightly soft and pliable.
2. Carefully cut open each pita pocket to create a pocket for filling.
3. Spread a generous amount of hummus inside each pita pocket.

4. Stuff each pocket with cucumber slices, bell pepper slices, shredded carrots, and spinach leaves.
5. Serve immediately and enjoy these delicious and nutritious stuffed pita pockets as a satisfying snack!

Nutrition Facts (per serving):

- Calories: 280
- Protein: 10g
- Fat: 8g
- Carbohydrates: 45g
- Fiber: 8g

Vegetable Sushi Rolls

Prep Time: 20 mins

Total Time: 20 mins

Servings: 2

Ingredients:

- 2 nori seaweed sheets
- 1 cup cooked sushi rice
- 1/2 cucumber, julienned
- 1/2 carrot, julienned
- 1/2 avocado, sliced
- 2 tablespoons rice vinegar
- 1 tablespoon soy sauce or tamari
- Pickled ginger and wasabi for serving (optional)

Directions:

1. Place a nori seaweed sheet on a bamboo sushi mat or clean kitchen towel.

2. Spread a thin layer of cooked sushi rice evenly over the nori sheet, leaving about 1 inch of space at the top.
3. Arrange cucumber, carrot, and avocado slices in a row along the bottom edge of the rice.
4. Using the sushi mat or towel, tightly roll up the nori sheet, pressing gently to seal the roll.
5. Repeat with the remaining ingredients to make the second sushi roll.
6. Use a sharp knife to slice each roll into bite-sized pieces.
7. Serve with soy sauce or tamari, pickled ginger, and wasabi on the side, if desired.
8. Enjoy these homemade vegetable sushi rolls as a healthy and flavorful snack!

Nutrition Facts (per serving - 1 roll):
- Calories: 220
- Protein: 5g
- Fat: 5g
- Carbohydrates: 40g
- Fiber: 5g

Crunchy Chickpea Snack

Prep Time: 5 mins

Total Time: 25 mins

Servings: 2

Ingredients:
- 1 can (15 oz) chickpeas, drained and rinsed
- 1 tablespoon olive oil

- 1 teaspoon paprika
- 1/2 teaspoon garlic powder
- 1/2 teaspoon cumin
- Salt and pepper to taste

Directions:

1. Preheat the oven to 400°F (200°C). Line a baking sheet with parchment paper.
2. Pat the chickpeas dry with a clean kitchen towel or paper towel.
3. In a mixing bowl, toss the chickpeas with olive oil, paprika, garlic powder, cumin, salt, and pepper until evenly coated.
4. Spread the chickpeas in a single layer on the prepared baking sheet.
5. Bake for 20-25 minutes, or until crispy and golden brown, stirring halfway through.
6. Remove from the oven and let cool before serving.
7. Enjoy these crunchy chickpeas as a satisfying and flavorful snack!

Nutrition Facts (per serving):

- Calories: 150
- Protein: 6g
- Fat: 7g
- Carbohydrates: 18g
- Fiber: 5g

Apple and Peanut Butter Rice Cakes

Prep Time: 5 mins

Total Time: 5 mins

Servings: 2

Ingredients:
- 2 rice cakes (whole grain or gluten-free)
- 2 tablespoons natural peanut butter
- 1 small apple, thinly sliced
- Cinnamon for sprinkling (optional)

Directions:
1. Spread a tablespoon of peanut butter onto each rice cake.
2. Arrange thinly sliced apple on top of the peanut butter.
3. Sprinkle with cinnamon, if desired.
4. Serve immediately and enjoy this simple and satisfying snack!

Nutrition Facts (per serving):
- Calories: 200
- Protein: 5g
- Fat: 10g
- Carbohydrates: 25g
- Fiber: 5g

Vegetable Crudité with Hummus

Prep Time: 10 mins

Total Time: 10 mins

Servings: 2

Ingredients:
- Assorted raw vegetables (such as baby carrots, cucumber sticks, bell pepper strips, cherry tomatoes)

- 1/2 cup hummus

Directions:

1. Wash and prepare the raw vegetables by cutting them into sticks or bite-sized pieces.
2. Arrange the vegetable crudité on a serving platter.
3. Serve with hummus for dipping.
4. Enjoy this colorful and nutritious snack!

Nutrition Facts (per serving):

- Calories: 150
- Protein: 6g
- Fat: 7g
- Carbohydrates: 20g
- Fiber: 7g

Quinoa and Black Bean Salad Cups

Prep Time: 10 mins

Total Time: 10 mins

Servings: 2

Ingredients:

- 1 cup cooked quinoa
- 1/2 cup black beans, drained and rinsed
- 1/4 cup diced bell pepper
- 1/4 cup diced cucumber
- 1/4 cup cherry tomatoes, halved
- 2 tablespoons chopped fresh cilantro
- Juice of 1 lime
- Salt and pepper to taste

Directions:

1. In a mixing bowl, combine cooked quinoa, black beans, diced bell pepper, diced cucumber, cherry tomatoes, chopped fresh cilantro, lime juice, salt, and pepper.
2. Stir until well combined.
3. Spoon the quinoa and black bean salad into small cups or bowls for serving.
4. Enjoy this refreshing and protein-packed snack!

Nutrition Facts (per serving):

- Calories: 200
- Protein: 8g
- Fat: 2g
- Carbohydrates: 38g
- Fiber: 7g

Banana Almond Butter Bites

Prep Time: 5 mins

Total Time: 5 mins

Servings: 2

Ingredients:

- 1 large banana, sliced
- 2 tablespoons almond butter
- 2 tablespoons granola

Directions:

1. Spread almond butter onto banana slices.
2. Sprinkle granola on top of almond butter.

3. Serve immediately and enjoy these delicious and satisfying bites!

Nutrition Facts (per serving):
- Calories: 180
- Protein: 4g
- Fat: 9g
- Carbohydrates: 22g
- Fiber: 3g

Zesty Cucumber Hummus Cups

Prep Time: 10 mins

Total Time: 10 mins

Servings: 2

Ingredients:
- 1 cucumber
- 1/2 cup hummus
- Cherry tomatoes, sliced
- Black olives, sliced
- Fresh parsley, chopped

Directions:
1. Wash the cucumber and cut it into thick slices, about 1 inch thick.
2. Use a melon baller or small spoon to scoop out some of the seeds from the center of each cucumber slice, creating a cup-like shape.
3. Fill each cucumber cup with a spoonful of hummus.

4. Top with sliced cherry tomatoes, black olives, and chopped parsley.
   5. Serve immediately and enjoy these refreshing and flavorful hummus cups!

Nutrition Facts (per serving):
- Calories: 100
- Protein: 5g
- Fat: 5g
- Carbohydrates: 10g
- Fiber: 4g

Crispy Baked Kale Chips

Prep Time: 10 mins

Total Time: 25 mins

Servings: 2

Ingredients:
- 1 bunch kale
- 1 tablespoon olive oil
- Salt and pepper to taste
- Optional: nutritional yeast, garlic powder, chili flakes

Directions:
   1. Preheat the oven to 300°F (150°C). Line a baking sheet with parchment paper.
   2. Wash the kale leaves and pat them dry with a clean kitchen towel or paper towel.
   3. Remove the tough stems from the kale leaves and tear the leaves into bite-sized pieces.

4. In a large mixing bowl, toss the kale pieces with olive oil, salt, pepper, and any optional seasonings of your choice.
5. Spread the seasoned kale pieces in a single layer on the prepared baking sheet.
6. Bake for 20-25 minutes, or until the kale chips are crispy and slightly golden brown, stirring halfway through.
7. Remove from the oven and let cool before serving.
8. Enjoy these crispy kale chips as a nutritious and satisfying snack!

Nutrition Facts (per serving):
- Calories: 80
- Protein: 5g
- Fat: 4g
- Carbohydrates: 10g
- Fiber: 3g

Sweet Potato Toasts with Almond Butter

Prep Time: 5 mins

Total Time: 15 mins

Servings: 2

Ingredients:
- 1 large sweet potato
- 2 tablespoons almond butter
- Optional toppings: sliced banana, chia seeds, cinnamon

Directions:
1. Wash the sweet potato and slice it lengthwise into thin slices, about 1/4 inch thick.

2. Toast the sweet potato slices in a toaster or toaster oven until they are cooked through and slightly crispy.
3. Spread a tablespoon of almond butter onto each sweet potato slice.
4. Top with sliced banana, chia seeds, and a sprinkle of cinnamon, if desired.
5. Serve immediately and enjoy these delicious and nutritious sweet potato toasts!

Nutrition Facts (per serving):
- Calories: 150
- Protein: 3g
- Fat: 8g
- Carbohydrates: 18g
- Fiber: 3g

Mango Salsa with Whole Grain Crackers

Prep Time: 10 mins

Total Time: 10 mins

Servings: 2

Ingredients:
- 1 ripe mango, diced
- 1/4 cup red onion, finely chopped
- 1/4 cup fresh cilantro, chopped
- 1 jalapeño pepper, seeded and finely chopped
- Juice of 1 lime
- Salt and pepper to taste
- Whole grain crackers for serving

Directions:
1. In a mixing bowl, combine diced mango, chopped red onion, chopped cilantro, chopped jalapeño pepper, lime juice, salt, and pepper. Stir until well combined.
2. Taste and adjust seasoning, if needed.
3. Serve the mango salsa with whole grain crackers for dipping.
4. Enjoy this vibrant and flavorful salsa as a delicious and wholesome snack!

Nutrition Facts (per serving):
- Calories: 120
- Protein: 2g
- Fat: 1g
- Carbohydrates: 30g
- Fiber: 4g

Quinoa-Stuffed Bell Pepper

Prep Time: 15 mins

Total Time: 45 mins

Servings: 2

Ingredients:
- 2 large bell peppers (any color), halved and seeds removed
- 1/2 cup cooked quinoa
- 1/2 cup cooked black beans, drained and rinsed
- 1/4 cup corn kernels
- 1/4 cup diced tomatoes
- 1/4 cup diced red onion
- 1/4 cup diced avocado

- 1/4 cup chopped fresh cilantro
- Juice of 1 lime
- Salt and pepper to taste
- Optional: shredded cheese, salsa

Directions:
1. Preheat the oven to 375°F (190°C). Place the halved bell peppers on a baking sheet.
2. In a mixing bowl, combine cooked quinoa, black beans, corn kernels, diced tomatoes, diced red onion, diced avocado, chopped cilantro, lime juice, salt, and pepper. Stir until well combined.
3. Spoon the quinoa mixture into each bell pepper half, pressing down gently to fill.
4. If desired, sprinkle shredded cheese on top of each stuffed bell pepper.
5. Bake for 25-30 minutes, or until the bell peppers are tender and the filling is heated through.
6. Remove from the oven and let cool slightly before serving.
7. Serve with salsa on the side, if desired.
8. Enjoy these flavorful and nutritious quinoa-stuffed bell peppers as a satisfying snack or light meal!

Nutrition Facts (per serving):
- Calories: 250
- Protein: 9g
- Fat: 6g
- Carbohydrates: 40g

- Fiber: 9g

Nutty Banana Oat Bars

Prep Time: 10 mins

Total Time: 30 mins

Servings: 8 bars

Ingredients:

- 2 ripe bananas, mashed
- 1 cup rolled oats
- 1/4 cup almond butter
- 1/4 cup chopped nuts (such as almonds, walnuts, or cashews)
- 1/4 cup dried fruit (such as raisins, cranberries, or apricots), chopped
- 1 tablespoon honey or maple syrup
- 1 teaspoon cinnamon
- Pinch of salt

Directions:

1. Preheat the oven to 350°F (175°C). Grease a baking dish or line it with parchment paper.
2. In a mixing bowl, combine mashed bananas, rolled oats, almond butter, chopped nuts, dried fruit, honey or maple syrup, cinnamon, and a pinch of salt. Stir until well combined.
3. Press the mixture evenly into the prepared baking dish.
4. Bake for 20-25 minutes, or until the bars are golden brown and firm to the touch.
5. Remove from the oven and let cool before slicing into bars.
6. Once cooled, cut into bars and store in an airtight container.

7. Enjoy these nutty banana oat bars as a wholesome and energizing snack!

Nutrition Facts (per serving):
- Calories: 150
- Protein: 4g
- Fat: 7g
- Carbohydrates: 20g
- Fiber: 3g

Roasted Chickpea Trail Mix

Prep Time: 10 mins

Total Time: 40 mins

Servings: 4

Ingredients:
- 1 can (15 oz) chickpeas, drained and rinsed
- 1 tablespoon olive oil
- 1 teaspoon ground cumin
- 1 teaspoon chili powder
- 1/2 teaspoon garlic powder
- 1/2 teaspoon paprika
- 1/4 teaspoon salt
- 1/4 cup dried cranberries
- 1/4 cup roasted almonds
- 1/4 cup pumpkin seeds
- 1/4 cup dark chocolate chips

Directions:

1. Preheat the oven to 400°F (200°C). Line a baking sheet with parchment paper.
2. Pat the chickpeas dry with a clean kitchen towel or paper towel.
3. In a mixing bowl, toss the chickpeas with olive oil, ground cumin, chili powder, garlic powder, paprika, and salt until evenly coated.
4. Spread the seasoned chickpeas in a single layer on the prepared baking sheet.
5. Roast for 30-35 minutes, stirring halfway through, until the chickpeas are crispy and golden brown.
6. Remove from the oven and let cool completely.
7. Once cooled, transfer the roasted chickpeas to a mixing bowl and add dried cranberries, roasted almonds, pumpkin seeds, and dark chocolate chips. Toss to combine.
8. Store the roasted chickpea trail mix in an airtight container for up to 1 week.
9. Enjoy this crunchy and flavorful trail mix as a satisfying snack on the go!

Nutrition Facts (per serving):
- Calories: 250
- Protein: 8g
- Fat: 10g
- Carbohydrates: 30g
- Fiber: 6g

Greek Yogurt Berry Parfait

Prep Time: 5 mins

Total Time: 5 mins

Servings: 2

Ingredients:

- 1 cup plain Greek yogurt
- 1/2 cup mixed berries (such as strawberries, blueberries, raspberries)
- 1/4 cup granola
- 1 tablespoon honey or maple syrup (optional)

Directions:

1. In a serving glass or bowl, layer the plain Greek yogurt, mixed berries, and granola.
2. Drizzle with honey or maple syrup, if using.
3. Repeat the layers until the glass or bowl is full.
4. Serve immediately and enjoy this creamy and nutritious Greek yogurt berry parfait!

Nutrition Facts (per serving):

- Calories: 180
- Protein: 15g
- Fat: 3g
- Carbohydrates: 30g
- Fiber: 3g

Stuffed Celery Sticks

Prep Time: 10 mins

Total Time: 10 mins

Servings: 2

Ingredients:
- 4 celery stalks, washed and trimmed
- 1/4 cup hummus
- 1/4 cup sliced almonds
- 1/4 cup dried cranberries

Directions:
1. Cut the celery stalks into halves or thirds, depending on their size.
2. Fill each celery stick with hummus.
3. Top with sliced almonds and dried cranberries.
4. Serve immediately and enjoy these crunchy and flavorful stuffed celery sticks!

Nutrition Facts (per serving):
- Calories: 120
- Protein: 4g
- Fat: 7g
- Carbohydrates: 12g
- Fiber: 4g

Turkey and Avocado Roll-Ups

Prep Time: 10 mins

Total Time: 10 mins

Servings: 2

Ingredients:
- 4 slices deli turkey breast
- 1 avocado, thinly sliced
- 1/4 cup baby spinach leaves

- 1 tablespoon hummus
- Salt and pepper to taste

Directions:

1. Lay out the turkey slices on a clean surface.
2. Spread a thin layer of hummus onto each turkey slice.
3. Place a few baby spinach leaves and avocado slices on top of each turkey slice.
4. Season with salt and pepper to taste.
5. Roll up each turkey slice tightly.
6. Secure with toothpicks if needed.
7. Serve immediately and enjoy these protein-packed turkey and avocado roll-ups!

Nutrition Facts (per serving):

- Calories: 180
- Protein: 15g
- Fat: 10g
- Carbohydrates: 6g
- Fiber: 4g

SMOOTHIE RECIPES

Berry Blast Smoothie

Prep Time: 5 mins

Total Time: 5 mins

Servings: 2 glasses

Ingredients:

- 1 cup frozen mixed berries (strawberries, blueberries, raspberries)
- 1/2 cup spinach leaves
- 1/2 ripe banana
- 1/2 cup unsweetened almond milk
- 1/2 cup plain Greek yogurt
- 1 tablespoon chia seeds
- 1 teaspoon honey (optional)

Directions:

1. Place all ingredients in a blender.
2. Blend until smooth and creamy.
3. If the consistency is too thick, add more almond milk.
4. Pour into glasses and serve immediately.

Nutritional Information (per serving):

- Calories: 150
- Protein: 8g
- Fat: 4g
- Carbohydrates: 23g
- Fiber: 6g

Tropical Paradise Smoothie

Prep Time: 5 mins

Total Time: 5 mins

Servings: 2 glasses

Ingredients:
- 1 cup frozen mango chunks
- 1/2 cup pineapple chunks
- 1/2 ripe banana
- 1/2 cup spinach leaves
- 1/2 cup coconut water
- 1/2 cup plain Greek yogurt
- 1 tablespoon shredded coconut

Directions:
1. Combine all ingredients in a blender.
2. Blend until smooth.
3. Add more coconut water if needed to reach desired consistency.
4. Pour into glasses and garnish with shredded coconut if desired.

Nutritional Information (per serving):
- Calories: 180
- Protein: 8g
- Fat: 3g
- Carbohydrates: 34g
- Fiber: 6g

Green Goddess Smoothie

Prep Time: 5 mins

Total Time: 5 mins

Servings: 2 glasses

Ingredients:

- 1 cup fresh spinach
- 1/2 ripe avocado
- 1/2 cucumber, peeled and chopped
- 1/2 cup coconut water
- 1/2 cup plain Greek yogurt
- Juice of 1/2 lime
- 1 tablespoon fresh mint leaves
- 1 teaspoon honey (optional)

Directions:

1. Combine all ingredients in a blender.
2. Blend until smooth and creamy.
3. Adjust sweetness with honey if desired.
4. Pour into glasses and serve immediately.

Nutritional Information (per serving):

- Calories: 160
- Protein: 8g
- Fat: 7g
- Carbohydrates: 18g
- Fiber: 6g

Protein Power Smoothie

Prep Time: 5 mins

Total Time: 5 mins

Servings: 2 glasses

Ingredients:

- 1 cup unsweetened almond milk
- 1/2 cup plain Greek yogurt
- 1 scoop vanilla protein powder
- 1/2 cup frozen strawberries
- 1/2 ripe banana
- 1 tablespoon almond butter
- 1 teaspoon honey (optional)

Directions:
1. Add all ingredients to a blender.
2. Blend until smooth and creamy.
3. Adjust sweetness with honey if needed.
4. Pour into glasses and enjoy immediately.

Nutritional Information (per serving):
- Calories: 240
- Protein: 25g
- Fat: 7g
- Carbohydrates: 20g
- Fiber: 4g

Coconut Kale Smoothie

Prep Time: 5 mins

Total Time: 5 mins

Servings: 2 glasses

Ingredients:
- 1 cup coconut water
- 1/2 cup coconut milk
- 1 cup kale leaves, stems removed

- 1/2 cup frozen pineapple chunks
- 1/2 frozen banana
- 1 tablespoon unsweetened shredded coconut

Directions:
1. Combine all ingredients in a blender.
2. Blend until smooth and creamy.
3. Add more coconut water if necessary to reach desired consistency.
4. Pour into glasses and serve immediately.

Nutritional Information (per serving):
- Calories: 150
- Protein: 3g
- Fat: 8g
- Carbohydrates: 20g
- Fiber: 4g

Tropical Green Smoothie

Prep Time: 5 mins

Total Time: 5 mins

Servings: 2 glasses

Ingredients:
- 1 cup frozen mango chunks
- 1/2 cup frozen pineapple chunks
- 1 cup spinach leaves
- 1/2 ripe banana
- 1 cup coconut water
- 1 tablespoon chia seeds

Directions:

1. Combine all ingredients in a blender.
2. Blend until smooth and creamy.
3. Add more coconut water if needed for desired consistency.
4. Pour into glasses and serve immediately.

Nutritional Information (per serving):

- Calories: 180
- Protein: 5g
- Fat: 5g
- Carbohydrates: 32g
- Fiber: 7g

Berry Spinach Smoothie

Prep Time: 5 mins

Total Time: 5 mins

Servings: 2 glasses

Ingredients:

- 1 cup frozen mixed berries (strawberries, blueberries, raspberries)
- 1 cup spinach leaves
- 1/2 ripe banana
- 1/2 cup almond milk
- 1 tablespoon flaxseeds
- 1 tablespoon honey (optional)

Directions:

1. Place all ingredients in a blender.
2. Blend until smooth.

3. Add more almond milk if necessary to reach desired consistency.
   4. Pour into glasses and serve immediately.

Nutritional Information (per serving):
- Calories: 160
- Protein: 4g
- Fat: 4g
- Carbohydrates: 30g
- Fiber: 7g

Creamy Avocado Smoothie

Prep Time: 5 mins

Total Time: 5 mins

Servings: 2 glasses

Ingredients:
- 1/2 avocado
- 1 cup spinach leaves
- 1/2 cucumber, peeled and chopped
- 1/2 cup coconut water
- Juice of 1/2 lime
- 1 tablespoon fresh mint leaves
- 1 teaspoon agave nectar (optional)

Directions:
1. Combine all ingredients in a blender.
2. Blend until smooth and creamy.
3. Adjust sweetness with agave nectar if desired.
4. Pour into glasses and serve immediately.

Nutritional Information (per serving):

- Calories: 120
- Protein: 3g
- Fat: 7g
- Carbohydrates: 14g
- Fiber: 6g

Peanut Butter Banana Smoothie

Prep Time: 5 mins

Total Time: 5 mins

Servings: 2 glasses

Ingredients:

- 1 ripe banana
- 2 tablespoons natural peanut butter
- 1 cup spinach leaves
- 1 cup unsweetened almond milk
- 1 tablespoon chia seeds
- 1 tablespoon honey (optional)

Directions:

1. Combine all ingredients in a blender.
2. Blend until smooth and creamy.
3. Add more almond milk if needed to reach desired consistency.
4. Pour into glasses and serve immediately.

Nutritional Information (per serving):

- Calories: 250
- Protein: 8g
- Fat: 15g

- Carbohydrates: 25g
- Fiber: 7g

Blueberry Almond Smoothie

Prep Time: 5 mins

Total Time: 5 mins

Servings: 2 glasses

Ingredients:

- 1 cup frozen blueberries
- 1 cup spinach leaves
- 1/2 cup almond milk
- 1/4 cup plain Greek yogurt
- 2 tablespoons almond butter
- 1 tablespoon honey (optional)

Directions:

1. Place all ingredients in a blender.
2. Blend until smooth and creamy.
3. Adjust sweetness with honey if desired.
4. Pour into glasses and serve immediately.

Nutritional Information (per serving):

- Calories: 230
- Protein: 8g
- Fat: 12g
- Carbohydrates: 25g
- Fiber: 6g

Berry Blast Smoothie

Prep Time: 5 mins
Total Time: 5 mins
Servings: 2 glasses

Ingredients:

- 1 cup frozen mixed berries (strawberries, blueberries, raspberries)
- 1/2 cup spinach leaves
- 1/2 ripe banana
- 1 cup almond milk
- 1 tablespoon chia seeds
- 1 teaspoon honey (optional)

Directions:

1. Place all ingredients in a blender.
2. Blend until smooth.
3. Add more almond milk if necessary to reach desired consistency.
4. Pour into glasses and serve immediately.

Nutritional Information (per serving):

- Calories: 180
- Protein: 4g
- Fat: 5g
- Carbohydrates: 30g
- Fiber: 8g

Green Goddess Smoothie

Prep Time: 5 mins
Total Time: 5 mins

Servings: 2 glasses

Ingredients:

- 1 cup spinach leaves
- 1/2 avocado
- 1/2 cucumber, peeled and chopped
- 1/2 cup coconut water
- Juice of 1/2 lime
- 1 tablespoon fresh mint leaves
- 1 teaspoon agave nectar (optional)

Directions:

1. Combine all ingredients in a blender.
2. Blend until smooth and creamy.
3. Adjust sweetness with agave nectar if desired.
4. Pour into glasses and serve immediately.

Nutritional Information (per serving):

- Calories: 120
- Protein: 3g
- Fat: 7g
- Carbohydrates: 14g
- Fiber: 6g

Tropical Paradise Smoothie

Prep Time: 5 mins

Total Time: 5 mins

Servings: 2 glasses

Ingredients:

- 1 cup frozen pineapple chunks

- 1/2 cup frozen mango chunks
- 1 cup spinach leaves
- 1/2 banana
- 1/2 cup coconut milk
- 1 tablespoon flaxseeds

Directions:
1. Combine all ingredients in a blender.
2. Blend until smooth.
3. Add more coconut milk if necessary for desired consistency.
4. Pour into glasses and serve immediately.

Nutritional Information (per serving):
- Calories: 200
- Protein: 4g
- Fat: 8g
- Carbohydrates: 30g
- Fiber: 6g

Creamy Berry Smoothie

Prep Time: 5 mins

Total Time: 5 mins

Servings: 2 glasses

Ingredients:
- 1 cup mixed frozen berries
- 1/2 cup Greek yogurt
- 1/2 cup almond milk
- 1 tablespoon almond butter
- 1 tablespoon honey (optional)

Directions:
1. Place all ingredients in a blender.
2. Blend until smooth and creamy.
3. Adjust sweetness with honey if desired.
4. Pour into glasses and serve immediately.

Nutritional Information (per serving):
- Calories: 230
- Protein: 9g
- Fat: 10g
- Carbohydrates: 29g
- Fiber: 6g

Chocolate Peanut Butter Smoothie

Prep Time: 5 mins

Total Time: 5 mins

Servings: 2 glasses

Ingredients:
- 1 ripe banana
- 2 tablespoons natural peanut butter
- 1 tablespoon cocoa powder
- 1 cup almond milk
- 1 tablespoon honey (optional)

Directions:
1. Combine all ingredients in a blender.
2. Blend until smooth and creamy.
3. Add more almond milk if needed to reach desired consistency.
4. Pour into glasses and serve immediately.

Nutritional Information (per serving):

- Calories: 280
- Protein: 8g
- Fat: 15g
- Carbohydrates: 33g
- Fiber: 7g

Green Detox Smoothie

Prep Time: 5 mins

Total Time: 5 mins

Servings: 2 glasses

Ingredients:

- 1 cup spinach
- 1/2 cup kale
- 1/2 cucumber, chopped
- 1/2 green apple, chopped
- 1/2 avocado
- Juice of 1 lemon
- 1 cup coconut water
- 1 tablespoon chia seeds
- Optional: 1 teaspoon honey or agave nectar

Directions:

1. Combine all ingredients in a blender.
2. Blend until smooth and creamy.
3. Taste and adjust sweetness with honey or agave nectar if desired.
4. Pour into glasses and serve immediately.

Nutritional Information (per serving):
- Calories: 150
- Protein: 5g
- Fat: 8g
- Carbohydrates: 18g
- Fiber: 7g

Berry Blast Smoothie

Prep Time: 5 mins

Total Time: 5 mins

Servings: 2 glasses

Ingredients:
- 1 cup frozen mixed berries (strawberries, blueberries, raspberries)
- 1/2 banana
- 1/2 cup spinach
- 1/2 cup almond milk
- 1 tablespoon flaxseeds
- Optional: 1 teaspoon honey or maple syrup

Directions:
1. Combine all ingredients in a blender.
2. Blend until smooth.
3. Adjust sweetness with honey or maple syrup if needed.
4. Pour into glasses and serve immediately.

Nutritional Information (per serving):
- Calories: 160
- Protein: 4g

- Fat: 6g
- Carbohydrates: 25g
- Fiber: 7g

Tropical Paradise Smoothie

Prep Time: 5 mins

Total Time: 5 mins

Servings: 2 glasses

Ingredients:

- 1/2 cup frozen pineapple chunks
- 1/2 cup frozen mango chunks
- 1/2 banana
- 1/2 cup coconut milk
- 1/2 cup spinach
- 1 tablespoon hemp seeds
- Optional: 1 teaspoon honey or agave nectar

Directions:

1. Combine all ingredients in a blender.
2. Blend until smooth.
3. Add honey or agave nectar for sweetness if desired.
4. Pour into glasses and serve immediately.

Nutritional Information (per serving):

- Calories: 220
- Protein: 4g
- Fat: 11g
- Carbohydrates: 29g
- Fiber: 5g

Creamy Peanut Butter Banana Smoothie

Prep Time: 5 mins

Total Time: 5 mins

Servings: 2 glasses

Ingredients:
- 1 banana
- 2 tablespoons natural peanut butter
- 1 cup almond milk
- 1/2 cup spinach
- 1 tablespoon chia seeds
- Optional: 1 teaspoon honey or maple syrup

Directions:
1. Combine all ingredients in a blender.
2. Blend until smooth and creamy.
3. Sweeten with honey or maple syrup if desired.
4. Pour into glasses and serve immediately.

Nutritional Information (per serving):
- Calories: 270
- Protein: 8g
- Fat: 15g
- Carbohydrates: 27g
- Fiber: 7g

Vanilla Almond Protein Smoothie

Prep Time: 5 mins

Total Time: 5 mins

Servings: 2 glasses

Ingredients:
- 1 cup unsweetened almond milk
- 1 scoop vanilla protein powder
- 1/2 banana
- 1 tablespoon almond butter
- 1/2 cup spinach
- Optional: 1 teaspoon honey or maple syrup

Directions:
1. Combine all ingredients in a blender.
2. Blend until smooth.
3. Sweeten with honey or maple syrup if desired.
4. Pour into glasses and serve immediately.

Nutritional Information (per serving):
- Calories: 240
- Protein: 22g
- Fat: 10g
- Carbohydrates: 17g
- Fiber: 4g

SEAFOOD RECIPES

Grilled Lemon Herb Salmon

Prep Time: 10 mins

Total Time: 20 mins

Servings: 4

Ingredients:

- 4 salmon fillets (about 6 oz each)
- 2 tablespoons olive oil
- 2 cloves garlic, minced
- 1 tablespoon fresh lemon juice
- 1 teaspoon lemon zest
- 1 teaspoon chopped fresh thyme
- Salt and pepper to taste
- Lemon wedges for serving
- Fresh parsley for garnish (optional)

Directions:

1. Preheat grill to medium-high heat.
2. In a small bowl, mix together olive oil, minced garlic, lemon juice, lemon zest, and chopped thyme.
3. Brush both sides of the salmon fillets with the lemon herb mixture and season with salt and pepper.
4. Place the salmon fillets on the grill and cook for about 4-5 minutes per side, or until cooked through and flaky.
5. Remove from the grill and serve hot with lemon wedges. Garnish with fresh parsley if desired.

Nutritional Information (per serving):

- Calories: 300
- Protein: 34g
- Fat: 18g
- Carbohydrates: 1g
- Fiber: 0g

Baked Lemon Garlic Shrimp

Prep Time: 10 mins

Total Time: 20 mins

Servings: 4

Ingredients:

- 1 lb large shrimp, peeled and deveined
- 2 tablespoons olive oil
- 3 cloves garlic, minced
- 2 tablespoons fresh lemon juice
- 1 teaspoon lemon zest
- 1 teaspoon dried oregano
- Salt and pepper to taste
- Fresh parsley for garnish
- Lemon wedges for serving

Directions:

1. Preheat oven to 400°F (200°C).
2. In a large bowl, combine olive oil, minced garlic, lemon juice, lemon zest, dried oregano, salt, and pepper.
3. Add the shrimp to the bowl and toss until evenly coated.
4. Transfer the shrimp to a baking dish in a single layer.

5. Bake in the preheated oven for 8-10 minutes, or until the shrimp are pink and cooked through.
6. Remove from the oven, garnish with fresh parsley, and serve with lemon wedges.

Nutritional Information (per serving):
- Calories: 180
- Protein: 24g
- Fat: 8g
- Carbohydrates: 3g
- Fiber: 0g

Seared Scallops with Garlic Butter

Prep Time: 10 mins
Total Time: 15 mins
Servings: 4

Ingredients:
- 1 lb large sea scallops
- 2 tablespoons unsalted butter
- 2 cloves garlic, minced
- Salt and pepper to taste
- Fresh parsley for garnish
- Lemon wedges for serving

Directions:
1. Pat the scallops dry with paper towels and season with salt and pepper on both sides.
2. Heat a large skillet over medium-high heat and add butter.

3. Once the butter has melted, add minced garlic to the skillet and cook for about 1 minute until fragrant.
4. Add the scallops to the skillet in a single layer, making sure not to overcrowd the pan. Cook for 2-3 minutes per side, or until golden brown and caramelized.
5. Remove the scallops from the skillet and transfer to a serving plate.
6. Garnish with fresh parsley and serve immediately with lemon wedges.

Nutritional Information (per serving):
- Calories: 160
- Protein: 19g
- Fat: 8g
- Carbohydrates: 2g
- Fiber: 0g

Grilled Shrimp Skewers

Prep Time: 15 mins

Total Time: 20 mins

Servings: 4

Ingredients:
- 1 lb large shrimp, peeled and deveined
- 2 tablespoons olive oil
- 2 cloves garlic, minced
- 1 tablespoon fresh lemon juice
- 1 teaspoon lemon zest
- 1 teaspoon paprika

- Salt and pepper to taste
- Wooden skewers, soaked in water for 30 minutes
- Lemon wedges for serving
- Fresh parsley for garnish

Directions:
1. Preheat grill to medium-high heat.
2. In a large bowl, combine olive oil, minced garlic, lemon juice, lemon zest, paprika, salt, and pepper.
3. Add the shrimp to the bowl and toss until evenly coated.
4. Thread the shrimp onto the soaked wooden skewers.
5. Grill the shrimp skewers for 2-3 minutes per side, or until they are pink and cooked through.
6. Remove from the grill and serve hot with lemon wedges. Garnish with fresh parsley if desired.

Nutritional Information (per serving):
- Calories: 180
- Protein: 22g
- Fat: 9g
- Carbohydrates: 2g
- Fiber: 0g

Pan-Seared Halibut with Lemon Herb Sauce

Prep Time: 10 mins

Total Time: 20 mins

Servings: 4

Ingredients:
- 4 halibut fillets (about 6 oz each)

- Salt and pepper to taste
- 2 tablespoons olive oil
- 2 tablespoons unsalted butter
- 2 cloves garlic, minced
- 2 tablespoons fresh lemon juice
- 1 teaspoon lemon zest
- 1 tablespoon chopped fresh parsley
- 1 tablespoon chopped fresh dill

Directions:

1. Season the halibut fillets with salt and pepper on both sides.
2. Heat olive oil in a large skillet over medium-high heat.
3. Add the halibut fillets to the skillet and cook for 3-4 minutes per side, or until golden brown and cooked through.
4. Remove the halibut from the skillet and transfer to a serving plate.
5. In the same skillet, melt butter over medium heat. Add minced garlic and cook for 1 minute until fragrant.
6. Stir in fresh lemon juice, lemon zest, chopped parsley, and chopped dill. Cook for another minute, then remove from heat.
7. Spoon the lemon herb sauce over the pan-seared halibut fillets.
8. Serve immediately with your choice of side dishes.

Nutritional Information (per serving):

- Calories: 250
- Protein: 30g
- Fat: 14g
- Carbohydrates: 1g

- Fiber: 0g

These seafood recipes are not only delicious but also suitable for individuals following an EPI diet, providing essential nutrients while being gentle on the digestive system. Enjoy these flavorful dishes as part of a balanced diet.

Cajun Grilled Shrimp Tacos

Prep Time: 15 mins

Total Time: 25 mins

Servings: 4

Ingredients:
- 1 lb large shrimp, peeled and deveined
- 2 tablespoons olive oil
- 2 teaspoons Cajun seasoning
- Salt and pepper to taste
- 8 small corn tortillas
- 1 cup shredded cabbage
- 1 avocado, sliced
- 1/4 cup diced tomatoes
- 1/4 cup diced red onions
- Lime wedges for serving
- Fresh cilantro for garnish

Directions:
1. Preheat grill to medium-high heat.
2. In a bowl, toss the shrimp with olive oil, Cajun seasoning, salt, and pepper until evenly coated.
3. Thread the seasoned shrimp onto skewers.

4. Grill the shrimp skewers for 2-3 minutes per side, or until they are pink and cooked through.
5. Warm the corn tortillas on the grill for about 30 seconds per side.
6. To assemble the tacos, place a few shrimp on each tortilla and top with shredded cabbage, sliced avocado, diced tomatoes, and red onions.
7. Serve the tacos hot with lime wedges on the side for squeezing. Garnish with fresh cilantro.

Nutritional Information (per serving):

- Calories: 280
- Protein: 22g
- Fat: 12g
- Carbohydrates: 24g
- Fiber: 6g

Baked Lemon Garlic Cod

Prep Time: 10 mins

Total Time: 20 mins

Servings: 4

Ingredients:

- 4 cod fillets (about 6 oz each)
- 2 tablespoons olive oil
- 3 cloves garlic, minced
- 2 tablespoons fresh lemon juice
- 1 teaspoon lemon zest
- 1 teaspoon dried parsley

- Salt and pepper to taste
- Lemon wedges for serving
- Fresh parsley for garnish

Directions:

1. Preheat oven to 400°F (200°C).
2. Place the cod fillets on a baking sheet lined with parchment paper.
3. In a small bowl, whisk together olive oil, minced garlic, lemon juice, lemon zest, dried parsley, salt, and pepper.
4. Drizzle the lemon garlic mixture over the cod fillets.
5. Bake in the preheated oven for 12-15 minutes, or until the cod is opaque and flakes easily with a fork.
6. Remove from the oven and serve hot with lemon wedges. Garnish with fresh parsley.

Nutritional Information (per serving):

- Calories: 220
- Protein: 26g
- Fat: 10g
- Carbohydrates: 2g
- Fiber: 0g

Coconut Shrimp Curry

Prep Time: 15 mins

Total Time: 30 mins

Servings: 4

Ingredients:

- 1 lb large shrimp, peeled and deveined

- 2 tablespoons coconut oil
- 1 onion, diced
- 3 cloves garlic, minced
- 1 tablespoon grated ginger
- 2 tablespoons curry powder
- 1 teaspoon ground turmeric
- 1 can (14 oz) coconut milk
- 1 cup vegetable broth
- 1 tablespoon fish sauce
- 2 cups fresh spinach
- Salt and pepper to taste
- Cooked rice for serving

Directions:

1. In a large skillet, heat coconut oil over medium heat. Add diced onion and cook until softened.
2. Add minced garlic and grated ginger to the skillet and cook for 1 minute until fragrant.
3. Stir in curry powder and ground turmeric, and cook for another minute.
4. Pour in coconut milk, vegetable broth, and fish sauce. Bring to a simmer.
5. Add shrimp to the skillet and cook for 5-7 minutes, or until the shrimp are pink and cooked through.
6. Stir in fresh spinach and cook until wilted. Season with salt and pepper to taste.
7. Serve the coconut shrimp curry hot over cooked rice.

Nutritional Information (per serving):
- Calories: 320
- Protein: 24g
- Fat: 21g
- Carbohydrates: 15g
- Fiber: 2g

Lemon Garlic Butter Scallops

Prep Time: 10 mins

Total Time: 15 mins

Servings: 4

Ingredients:
- 1 lb large sea scallops
- Salt and pepper to taste
- 2 tablespoons unsalted butter
- 3 cloves garlic, minced
- 2 tablespoons fresh lemon juice
- 1 teaspoon lemon zest
- 1 tablespoon chopped fresh parsley

Directions:
1. Pat the scallops dry with paper towels and season with salt and pepper on both sides.
2. Heat a large skillet over medium-high heat and add butter.
3. Once the butter has melted, add minced garlic to the skillet and cook for 1 minute until fragrant.

4. Add the scallops to the skillet in a single layer and cook for 2-3 minutes per side, or until they are golden brown and opaque in the center.
5. Drizzle fresh lemon juice over the scallops and sprinkle with lemon zest and chopped parsley.
6. Remove from heat and serve the lemon garlic butter scallops immediately.

Nutritional Information (per serving):
- Calories: 180
- Protein: 20g
- Fat: 9g
- Carbohydrates: 4g
- Fiber: 0g

Grilled Salmon with Dill Sauce

Prep Time: 10 mins

Total Time: 20 mins

Servings: 4

Ingredients:
- 4 salmon fillets (about 6 oz each)
- 2 tablespoons olive oil
- Salt and pepper to taste
- 1/4 cup Greek yogurt
- 2 tablespoons chopped fresh dill
- 1 tablespoon lemon juice
- 1 teaspoon lemon zest
- 1 clove garlic, minced

Directions:
1. Preheat grill to medium-high heat.
2. Brush salmon fillets with olive oil and season with salt and pepper.
3. Grill the salmon fillets for 4-5 minutes per side, or until they are cooked through and flake easily with a fork.
4. In a small bowl, mix together Greek yogurt, chopped fresh dill, lemon juice, lemon zest, and minced garlic to make the dill sauce.
5. Serve the grilled salmon hot with a dollop of dill sauce on top.

Nutritional Information (per serving):
- Calories: 320
- Protein: 28g
- Fat: 20g
- Carbohydrates: 2g
- Fiber: 0g

Grilled Lemon Herb Salmon

Prep Time: 10 mins

Total Time: 20 mins

Servings: 4

Ingredients:
- 4 salmon fillets (6 oz each)
- 2 tablespoons olive oil
- 2 cloves garlic, minced
- 1 tablespoon fresh lemon juice
- 1 teaspoon lemon zest

- 1 teaspoon chopped fresh thyme
- Salt and pepper to taste
- Lemon wedges for serving
- Fresh parsley for garnish

Directions:
1. Preheat grill to medium-high heat.
2. In a small bowl, whisk together olive oil, minced garlic, lemon juice, lemon zest, chopped thyme, salt, and pepper.
3. Brush the mixture over the salmon fillets, coating evenly.
4. Place the salmon fillets on the grill and cook for 4-5 minutes per side, or until the fish flakes easily with a fork.
5. Remove from the grill and serve hot with lemon wedges. Garnish with fresh parsley.

Nutritional Information (per serving):
- Calories: 300
- Protein: 28g
- Fat: 18g
- Carbohydrates: 2g
- Fiber: 0g

Lemon Garlic Shrimp Pasta

Prep Time: 15 mins

Total Time: 25 mins

Servings: 4

Ingredients:
- 8 oz whole wheat pasta
- 1 lb large shrimp, peeled and deveined

- 2 tablespoons olive oil
- 4 cloves garlic, minced
- 2 tablespoons fresh lemon juice
- 1 teaspoon lemon zest
- 1/4 cup chopped fresh parsley
- Salt and pepper to taste
- Grated Parmesan cheese for serving

Directions:

1. Cook the pasta according to package instructions until al dente. Drain and set aside.
2. In a large skillet, heat olive oil over medium heat. Add minced garlic and cook until fragrant.
3. Add the shrimp to the skillet and cook for 2-3 minutes per side, or until pink and cooked through.
4. Stir in fresh lemon juice, lemon zest, chopped parsley, salt, and pepper.
5. Add the cooked pasta to the skillet and toss until well coated with the shrimp and sauce.
6. Serve hot with grated Parmesan cheese on top.

Nutritional Information (per serving):

- Calories: 380
- Protein: 30g
- Fat: 10g
- Carbohydrates: 40g
- Fiber: 6g

Baked Lemon Dill Cod

Prep Time: 10 mins

Total Time: 20 mins

Servings: 4

Ingredients:

- 4 cod fillets (6 oz each)
- 2 tablespoons olive oil
- 2 cloves garlic, minced
- 2 tablespoons fresh lemon juice
- 1 teaspoon lemon zest
- 1 tablespoon chopped fresh dill
- Salt and pepper to taste
- Lemon wedges for serving

Directions:

1. Preheat oven to 400°F (200°C).
2. Place the cod fillets on a baking sheet lined with parchment paper.
3. In a small bowl, whisk together olive oil, minced garlic, lemon juice, lemon zest, chopped dill, salt, and pepper.
4. Brush the mixture over the cod fillets, coating evenly.
5. Bake in the preheated oven for 12-15 minutes, or until the fish is opaque and flakes easily with a fork.
6. Serve hot with lemon wedges on the side.

Nutritional Information (per serving):

- Calories: 240
- Protein: 30g
- Fat: 10g

- Carbohydrates: 2g
- Fiber: 0g

Garlic Butter Scallops

Prep Time: 10 mins

Total Time: 15 mins

Servings: 4

Ingredients:
- 1 lb large sea scallops
- 2 tablespoons unsalted butter
- 2 cloves garlic, minced
- 1 tablespoon chopped fresh parsley
- Salt and pepper to taste
- Lemon wedges for serving

Directions:
1. Pat the scallops dry with paper towels and season with salt and pepper.
2. Heat a large skillet over medium-high heat and add butter.
3. Once the butter has melted, add minced garlic to the skillet and cook for 1 minute until fragrant.
4. Add the scallops to the skillet in a single layer and cook for 2-3 minutes per side, or until they are golden brown and opaque in the center.
5. Sprinkle chopped fresh parsley over the scallops and serve hot with lemon wedges.

Nutritional Information (per serving):
- Calories: 160

- Protein: 20g
- Fat: 8g
- Carbohydrates: 2g
- Fiber: 0g

Lemon Herb Tilapia

Prep Time: 10 mins

Total Time: 20 mins

Servings: 4

Ingredients:

- 4 tilapia fillets (6 oz each)
- 2 tablespoons olive oil
- 2 cloves garlic, minced
- 2 tablespoons fresh lemon juice
- 1 teaspoon lemon zest
- 1 tablespoon chopped fresh parsley
- Salt and pepper to taste

Directions:

1. Preheat oven to 400°F (200°C).
2. Place the tilapia fillets on a baking sheet lined with parchment paper.
3. In a small bowl, whisk together olive oil, minced garlic, lemon juice, lemon zest, chopped parsley, salt, and pepper.
4. Brush the mixture over the tilapia fillets, coating evenly.
5. Bake in the preheated oven for 12-15 minutes, or until the fish is opaque and flakes easily with a fork.
6. Serve hot with additional lemon wedges if desired.

Nutritional Information (per serving):

- Calories: 180
- Protein: 26g
- Fat: 8g
- Carbohydrates: 2g
- Fiber: 0g

Lemon Garlic Grilled Shrimp

Prep Time: 10 mins

Total Time: 15 mins

Servings: 4

Ingredients:

- 1 lb large shrimp, peeled and deveined
- 2 cloves garlic, minced
- 2 tablespoons olive oil
- 1 tablespoon fresh lemon juice
- 1 teaspoon lemon zest
- 1 teaspoon chopped fresh parsley
- Salt and pepper to taste
- Lemon wedges for serving

Directions:

1. Preheat grill to medium-high heat.
2. In a bowl, combine minced garlic, olive oil, lemon juice, lemon zest, chopped parsley, salt, and pepper.
3. Add the shrimp to the bowl and toss until evenly coated.
4. Thread the shrimp onto skewers.

5. Grill the shrimp for 2-3 minutes per side until pink and cooked through.
6. Serve hot with lemon wedges on the side.

Nutritional Information (per serving):
- Calories: 180
- Protein: 25g
- Fat: 8g
- Carbohydrates: 2g
- Fiber: 0g

Baked Salmon with Dill

Prep Time: 10 mins

Total Time: 20 mins

Servings: 4

Ingredients:
- 4 salmon fillets (6 oz each)
- 2 tablespoons olive oil
- 2 cloves garlic, minced
- 1 tablespoon fresh lemon juice
- 1 teaspoon lemon zest
- 1 tablespoon chopped fresh dill
- Salt and pepper to taste
- Lemon wedges for serving

Directions:
1. Preheat oven to 400°F (200°C).
2. Place the salmon fillets on a baking sheet lined with parchment paper.

3. In a bowl, whisk together olive oil, minced garlic, lemon juice, lemon zest, chopped dill, salt, and pepper.
4. Brush the mixture over the salmon fillets, coating evenly.
5. Bake in the preheated oven for 12-15 minutes until the salmon flakes easily with a fork.
6. Serve hot with lemon wedges on the side.

Nutritional Information (per serving):
- Calories: 320
- Protein: 35g
- Fat: 18g
- Carbohydrates: 2g
- Fiber: 0g

Garlic Butter Lobster Tails

- **Prep Time:** 10 mins
- **Total Time:** 20 mins
- **Servings:** 4

Ingredients:
- 4 lobster tails
- 4 tablespoons unsalted butter
- 4 cloves garlic, minced
- 1 tablespoon chopped fresh parsley
- Salt and pepper to taste
- Lemon wedges for serving

Directions:
1. Preheat oven to 375°F (190°C).

2. Use kitchen shears to cut the top of each lobster tail shell lengthwise.
3. In a microwave-safe bowl, melt the butter and stir in minced garlic and chopped parsley.
4. Brush the garlic butter mixture over the lobster tails.
5. Place the lobster tails on a baking sheet and bake for 12-15 minutes until the lobster meat is opaque and white.
6. Serve hot with lemon wedges on the side.

Nutritional Information (per serving):
- Calories: 230
- Protein: 25g
- Fat: 14g
- Carbohydrates: 1g
- Fiber: 0g

Tuna Salad Lettuce Wraps

Prep Time: 15 mins

Total Time: 15 mins

Servings: 4

Ingredients:
- 2 cans (5 oz each) tuna, drained
- 1/4 cup mayonnaise
- 2 tablespoons chopped celery
- 2 tablespoons chopped red onion
- 1 tablespoon lemon juice
- Salt and pepper to taste
- Lettuce leaves for wrapping

Directions:

1. In a bowl, combine drained tuna, mayonnaise, chopped celery, chopped red onion, lemon juice, salt, and pepper.
2. Mix until well combined.
3. Spoon the tuna salad onto lettuce leaves.
4. Wrap the lettuce around the filling to form wraps.
5. Serve immediately.

Nutritional Information (per serving):

- Calories: 180
- Protein: 20g
- Fat: 10g
- Carbohydrates: 2g
- Fiber: 1g

Grilled Swordfish with Mango Salsa

Prep Time: 15 mins

Total Time: 25 mins

Servings: 4

Ingredients:

- 4 swordfish steaks (6 oz each)
- 2 tablespoons olive oil
- Salt and pepper to taste

Mango Salsa:

- 1 mango, peeled and diced
- 1/4 cup diced red bell pepper
- 2 tablespoons chopped fresh cilantro
- 1 tablespoon lime juice

- 1 tablespoon finely chopped red onion
- Salt and pepper to taste

Directions:
1. Preheat grill to medium-high heat.
2. Rub swordfish steaks with olive oil and season with salt and pepper.
3. Grill swordfish for 4-5 minutes per side until cooked through and grill marks appear.
4. In a bowl, combine diced mango, diced red bell pepper, chopped cilantro, lime juice, chopped red onion, salt, and pepper to make the salsa.
5. Serve grilled swordfish topped with mango salsa.

Nutritional Information (per serving):
- Calories: 280
- Protein: 30g
- Fat: 10g
- Carbohydrates: 15g
- Fiber: 2g

GROCERY SHOPPING AND MEAL PREPARATION TIPS

Effective grocery shopping and meal preparation are essential components of a successful EPI Diet plan. In this chapter, we'll explore strategies for stocking your pantry for success, meal prepping for busy endomorphs, and smart shopping strategies to help you stay on track with your nutrition goals.

Stocking Your Pantry for Success

Stocking your pantry with nutritious staples is the first step towards making healthy eating easier and more convenient. By having the right ingredients on hand, you can quickly and easily prepare meals that align with the principles of the EPI Diet. Here are some essential items to include in your pantry:

- **Whole Grains**: Opt for whole grains such as brown rice, quinoa, oats, and whole wheat pasta. These complex carbohydrates provide sustained energy and are rich in fiber, vitamins, and minerals.

- **Lean Proteins**: Choose lean sources of protein such as chicken breast, turkey, fish, tofu, and legumes. Protein is essential for muscle growth and repair, and it also helps to promote feelings of fullness and satisfaction.

- **Healthy Fats**: Include healthy fats such as avocados, nuts, seeds, and olive oil in your pantry. These fats are important for heart health, hormone balance, and brain function.

- **Fruits and Vegetables**: Stock up on a variety of fresh, frozen, and canned fruits and vegetables. These colorful foods are rich in vitamins, minerals, and antioxidants, and they add flavor and texture to meals.
- **Herbs and Spices**: Herbs and spices are essential for adding flavor to your dishes without adding extra calories or sodium. Keep a variety of herbs and spices on hand, such as basil, oregano, garlic, cinnamon, and cumin.
- **Healthy Snacks**: Choose nutritious snacks such as Greek yogurt, hummus, fresh fruit, and raw nuts and seeds. These snacks provide a quick and convenient way to satisfy hunger between meals without derailing your diet.
- **Whole Food Condiments**: Opt for whole food condiments such as mustard, salsa, and vinegar-based dressings instead of high-calorie, processed condiments like mayonnaise or ketchup.

By keeping these pantry staples on hand, you'll have everything you need to whip up healthy and delicious meals that support your EPI Diet goals.

Meal Prepping for Busy Endomorphs

Meal prepping is a game-changer for busy endomorphs who struggle to find the time and energy to cook healthy meals during the week. By spending a little time upfront to prepare meals and snacks in advance, you can save time, money, and stress throughout the week. Here are some meal prepping tips for busy endomorphs:

- **Plan Your Meals**: Take some time at the beginning of the week to plan out your meals and snacks. Choose recipes that are simple, nutritious, and easy to prepare in large batches.
- **Batch Cooking**: Cook large batches of staple foods such as grains, proteins, and vegetables that can be used in multiple meals throughout the week. Roast a tray of vegetables, grill a batch of chicken breasts, or cook a pot of quinoa to have on hand for quick and easy meals.
- **Portion Control**: Once your meals are cooked, portion them out into individual containers for easy grab-and-go meals throughout the week. This helps to prevent overeating and ensures that you have balanced meals ready to eat whenever hunger strikes.
- **Stock Up on Grab-and-Go Snacks**: Prepare healthy snacks such as cut-up fruits and vegetables, Greek yogurt cups, and homemade energy balls to have on hand for quick and convenient snacks during the week.
- **Use Time-Saving Kitchen Tools**: Invest in time-saving kitchen tools such as a slow cooker, Instant Pot, or food processor to help streamline meal prep and make cooking easier and more efficient.
- **Make Use of Leftovers**: Don't let leftovers go to waste! Incorporate leftover ingredients into new meals or repurpose them into creative dishes to prevent food waste and save time and money.

By incorporating meal prepping into your routine, you can simplify your meal planning process, save time during the week, and ensure that you have nutritious meals and snacks readily available to support your EPI Diet goals.

Smart Shopping Strategies

Smart shopping strategies are essential for making healthy choices at the grocery store and staying on track with your nutrition goals. By planning ahead and making thoughtful choices, you can stock your kitchen with nutritious foods that support your health and well-being. Here are some smart shopping strategies to help you make the most of your grocery trips:

- **Make a List**: Before heading to the grocery store, make a list of the items you need based on your meal plan for the week. Stick to your list to avoid impulse purchases and ensure that you only buy what you need.
- **Shop the Perimeter**: When navigating the aisles of the grocery store, focus on shopping the perimeter where you'll find fresh produce, lean proteins, and whole foods. This is where the majority of nutrient-dense foods are located, while processed and packaged foods are typically found in the center aisles.
- **Read Labels**: Take the time to read food labels and ingredients lists to make informed choices about the foods you're buying. Look for products with minimal ingredients and avoid those with added sugars, artificial flavors, and preservatives.
- **Buy in Bulk**: Consider buying staple items such as grains, beans, and nuts in bulk to save money and reduce packaging waste. Just be sure to store them properly in airtight containers to maintain freshness.

- **Choose Seasonal Produce**: Opt for seasonal fruits and vegetables when possible, as they tend to be fresher, tastier, and more affordable than out-of-season produce. Plus, eating seasonally supports local farmers and reduces your carbon footprint.
- **Shop with a Full Stomach**: Avoid shopping on an empty stomach, as you're more likely to make impulse purchases and choose less nutritious foods when hungry. Instead, try to shop after a meal or snack when you're feeling satisfied.
- **Compare Prices**: Take the time to compare prices and look for sales and discounts on your favorite items. Consider purchasing generic or store-brand products to save money without sacrificing quality.

By implementing these smart shopping strategies, you can make healthier choices at the grocery store and set yourself up for success on the EPI Diet. Remember to plan ahead, stick to your list, and prioritize nutrient-dense foods to support your health and well-being.

EXERCISE AND LIFESTYLE RECOMMENDATIONS

Incorporating regular exercise and adopting healthy lifestyle habits are crucial components of a holistic approach to health and wellness, especially for individuals with an endomorphic body type. In this chapter, we'll explore the importance of exercise for endomorphs, recommended workouts tailored to their needs, and tips for managing stress and improving sleep.

Exercise is not only essential for physical health but also plays a significant role in supporting mental well-being and overall quality of life. For endomorphs, who may have a tendency to store excess fat and struggle with weight management, exercise is particularly important for boosting metabolism, burning calories, and maintaining lean muscle mass.

Importance of Exercise for Endomorphs

Regular exercise offers a multitude of benefits for individuals with an endomorphic body type. Here are some key reasons why exercise is important for endomorphs:

- **Boosts Metabolism**: Endomorphs often have a slower metabolism compared to other body types, which can make it more challenging to lose weight or maintain a healthy weight. Regular exercise helps to boost metabolism, increase calorie expenditure, and support weight management efforts.
- **Burns Calories**: Exercise is an effective way to burn calories and create a calorie deficit, which is necessary for weight loss.

By incorporating regular physical activity into their routine, endomorphs can achieve a healthy balance between energy intake and expenditure and promote sustainable weight loss.

- **Builds Lean Muscle Mass**: Strength training, in particular, is beneficial for endomorphs as it helps to build lean muscle mass, which in turn increases metabolism and calorie burn. Including strength training exercises in your workout routine can help to sculpt and tone your body while also improving strength and overall fitness.
- **Improves Insulin Sensitivity**: Endomorphs may have a tendency to experience insulin resistance, which can lead to fluctuations in blood sugar levels and cravings for sugary or high-carbohydrate foods. Regular exercise helps to improve insulin sensitivity, making it easier to regulate blood sugar levels and manage cravings.
- **Supports Mental Health**: Exercise is not only beneficial for physical health but also plays a crucial role in supporting mental well-being. Physical activity releases endorphins, neurotransmitters that help to reduce stress, boost mood, and improve overall mental health and resilience.

Overall, incorporating regular exercise into your routine is essential for achieving and maintaining a healthy weight, supporting metabolic health, and improving overall well-being, especially for individuals with an endomorphic body type.

Recommended Workouts for Endomorphs

When it comes to choosing workouts for endomorphs, it's important to focus on activities that support weight management, promote muscle growth, and improve overall fitness. Here are some recommended workouts tailored to the needs of endomorphs:

- **Strength Training**: Strength training should be a cornerstone of any workout routine for endomorphs. Focus on compound exercises that target multiple muscle groups simultaneously, such as squats, deadlifts, lunges, push-ups, and rows. Aim to include strength training exercises at least two to three times per week, with a mix of upper body, lower body, and core exercises.
- **Cardiovascular Exercise**: Cardiovascular exercise is important for burning calories, improving cardiovascular health, and boosting overall fitness. Endomorphs may benefit from a mix of moderate-intensity steady-state cardio (such as brisk walking, cycling, or swimming) and high-intensity interval training (HIIT) to maximize calorie burn and metabolic efficiency.
- **Flexibility and Mobility Work**: Don't forget to include flexibility and mobility work in your workout routine to improve joint health, range of motion, and overall flexibility. Incorporate dynamic stretches, yoga, or Pilates into your routine to help prevent injury and improve functional movement patterns.
- **Active Recreation**: Incorporating activities you enjoy into your routine can help you stay motivated and make exercise feel less like a chore. Whether it's hiking, dancing, playing sports, or

gardening, find activities that bring you joy and make them a regular part of your routine.
- **Consistency and Progression**: Regardless of the type of workout you choose, consistency is key. Aim to exercise most days of the week, with a mix of different types of workouts to keep things interesting and prevent boredom. As you become fitter and stronger, gradually increase the intensity, duration, or frequency of your workouts to continue challenging your body and making progress towards your goals.

By incorporating a variety of workouts into your routine and focusing on strength training, cardiovascular exercise, flexibility, and consistency, you can maximize the benefits of exercise and support your health and fitness goals as an endomorph.

Stress Management and Sleep Tips

In addition to exercise, managing stress and prioritizing sleep are important components of a healthy lifestyle for endomorphs. Chronic stress and inadequate sleep can have negative effects on metabolism, appetite regulation, and overall well-being, making it more challenging to achieve and maintain a healthy weight. Here are some tips for managing stress and improving sleep:

- **Practice Stress-Relief Techniques**: Incorporate stress-relief techniques such as deep breathing, meditation, yoga, or tai chi into your daily routine to help reduce stress levels and promote relaxation. Taking time for yourself to unwind and de-stress can have a profound impact on your physical and mental well-being.

- **Stay Active**: Regular physical activity is not only beneficial for physical health but also plays a crucial role in managing stress and improving mood. Find activities you enjoy and make them a regular part of your routine to help relieve stress and boost your mood.
- **Prioritize Sleep**: Aim for seven to nine hours of quality sleep per night to support overall health and well-being. Establish a regular sleep schedule, create a relaxing bedtime routine, and create a sleep-friendly environment by keeping your bedroom cool, dark, and quiet.
- **Limit Caffeine and Screen Time**: Avoid consuming caffeine or using electronic devices close to bedtime, as these can interfere with sleep quality and make it more difficult to fall asleep. Instead, opt for calming activities such as reading, listening to music, or taking a warm bath before bed.
- **Manage Time Wisely**: Poor time management can contribute to stress and sleep disturbances. Take steps to prioritize tasks, set realistic goals, and delegate responsibilities when necessary to avoid feeling overwhelmed and improve work-life balance.

MEAL PLAN

Day 1
- **Breakfast:** Green Detox Smoothie
- **Lunch:** Berry Blast Smoothie
- **Dinner:** Grilled chicken Caesar salad with whole grain croutons

Day 2
- **Breakfast:** Tropical Paradise Smoothie
- **Lunch:** Creamy Peanut Butter Banana Smoothie
- **Dinner:** Baked salmon with quinoa tabbouleh and roasted carrots

Day 3
- **Breakfast:** Vanilla Almond Protein Smoothie
- **Lunch:** Green Detox Smoothie
- **Dinner:** Lentil soup with whole wheat bread and mixed greens salad

Day 4
- **Breakfast:** Berry Blast Smoothie
- **Lunch:** Tropical Paradise Smoothie
- **Dinner:** Spaghetti squash with marinara sauce and turkey meatballs

Day 5
- **Breakfast:** Creamy Peanut Butter Banana Smoothie
- **Lunch:** Vanilla Almond Protein Smoothie

- **Dinner:** Grilled shrimp tacos with avocado salsa and black bean salad

Day 6
- **Breakfast:** Green Detox Smoothie
- **Lunch:** Berry Blast Smoothie
- **Dinner:** Baked chicken thighs with sweet potato fries and steamed broccoli

Day 7
- **Breakfast:** Tropical Paradise Smoothie
- **Lunch:** Creamy Peanut Butter Banana Smoothie
- **Dinner:** Quinoa stuffed bell peppers with side salad

Day 8
- **Breakfast:** Vanilla Almond Protein Smoothie
- **Lunch:** Green Detox Smoothie
- Dinner: Beef and vegetable kebabs with couscous

Day 9
- **Breakfast:** Berry Blast Smoothie
- **Lunch:** Tropical Paradise Smoothie
- **Dinner:** Baked tilapia with wild rice pilaf and roasted Brussels sprouts

Day 10
- **Breakfast:** Creamy Peanut Butter Banana Smoothie
- **Lunch:** Vanilla Almond Protein Smoothie
- **Dinner:** Vegetarian lasagna with garlic bread and Caesar salad

Day 11
- **Breakfast:** Green Detox Smoothie
- **Lunch:** Berry Blast Smoothie
- **Dinner:** Grilled steak salad with mixed greens, tomatoes, and balsamic vinaigrette

Day 12
- **Breakfast:** Green Detox Smoothie
- **Lunch:** Berry Blast Smoothie
- **Dinner:** Grilled chicken with steamed vegetables

Day 13
- **Breakfast:** Tropical Paradise Smoothie
- **Lunch:** Creamy Peanut Butter Banana Smoothie
- **Dinner:** Baked salmon with quinoa and roasted vegetables

Day 14
- **Breakfast:** Vanilla Almond Protein Smoothie
- **Lunch:** Green Detox Smoothie
- **Dinner:** Stir-fried tofu with brown rice and mixed greens salad

Day 15
- **Breakfast:** Berry Blast Smoothie
- **Lunch:** Tropical Paradise Smoothie
- **Dinner:** Grilled shrimp skewers with cauliflower rice and sautéed spinach

Day 16
- **Breakfast:** Creamy Peanut Butter Banana Smoothie

- **Lunch:** Vanilla Almond Protein Smoothie
- **Dinner:** Baked chicken breast with sweet potato mash and steamed broccoli

Day 17

- **Breakfast:** Green Detox Smoothie
- **Lunch:** Berry Blast Smoothie
- **Dinner:** Pan-seared tilapia with quinoa pilaf and roasted asparagus

Day 18

- **Breakfast:** Tropical Paradise Smoothie
- **Lunch:** Creamy Peanut Butter Banana Smoothie
- **Dinner:** Vegetarian chili with cornbread and mixed greens salad

Day 19

- **Breakfast:** Vanilla Almond Protein Smoothie
- **Lunch:** Green Detox Smoothie
- **Dinner:** Grilled steak with roasted potatoes and sautéed kale

Day 20

- **Breakfast:** Berry Blast Smoothie
- **Lunch:** Tropical Paradise Smoothie
- **Dinner:** Baked cod with wild rice and steamed green beans

Day 21

- **Breakfast:** Creamy Peanut Butter Banana Smoothie
- **Lunch:** Vanilla Almond Protein Smoothie

- **Dinner:** Vegetable stir-fry with tofu and brown rice

CONCLUSION

In conclusion, we have explored various aspects of the EPI Diet, including understanding endomorphic body types, the principles of the diet, customizing meal plans, grocery shopping and meal preparation tips, exercise recommendations, and lifestyle strategies. Throughout this journey, it's become evident that achieving optimal health and wellness as an endomorph requires a multifaceted approach that encompasses nutrition, exercise, and lifestyle habits.

The EPI Diet offers a holistic framework for addressing the unique challenges faced by endomorphs, providing practical strategies for nourishing the body, supporting metabolism, and promoting sustainable weight loss. By focusing on balanced nutrition, portion control, and regular physical activity, individuals can harness the power of the EPI Diet to achieve their health and fitness goals while improving overall well-being.

Stocking your pantry with nutritious staples, meal prepping for convenience, and adopting smart shopping strategies are essential components of the EPI Diet that facilitate adherence to healthy eating habits. By planning ahead, making thoughtful choices at the grocery store, and preparing meals in advance, individuals can set themselves up for success and make healthier choices more accessible in their daily lives.

Incorporating regular exercise into your routine is paramount for endomorphs, as it not only supports weight management and metabolic health but also promotes mental well-being and overall quality of life. From strength training to cardiovascular exercise to flexibility work, finding activities that you enjoy and making them a regular part of your routine is key to long-term success.

Furthermore, prioritizing stress management and sleep hygiene are crucial components of a healthy lifestyle for endomorphs. By practicing stress-relief techniques, prioritizing sleep, and managing time wisely, individuals can reduce stress levels, improve sleep quality, and support overall health and well-being.

As we reflect on the principles and strategies discussed throughout this journey, let us remember the words of Hippocrates, the father of medicine, who famously said, "Let food be thy medicine and medicine be thy food." This timeless wisdom serves as a reminder of the profound impact that nutrition and lifestyle habits can have on our health and well-being. By making informed choices and prioritizing self-care, we have the power to transform our lives and achieve our full potential.

In closing, let us embrace the journey towards optimal health and wellness with enthusiasm and determination. With the knowledge and tools provided by the EPI Diet, we can embark on a path of self-discovery, empowerment, and transformation. Remember, every small step we take towards better health is a victory worth celebrating. So let us continue to nourish our bodies, move with purpose, and cultivate habits that support our well-being, one day at a time. As the saying goes, "Health is not just about being better, it's about being your best self."

www.ingramcontent.com/pod-product-compliance
Lightning Source LLC
Chambersburg PA
CBHW052155220526
45471CB00004B/1695